100 WAYS TO LIVE TO 100

People's Medical Society Books
Currently Available from Wings Books

Blood Pressure: Questions You Have ... Answers You Need

Dial 800 For Health

Getting The Most For Your Medical Dollar

150 Ways To Be A Savvy Medical Consumer

Take This Book To The Hospital With You

Take This Book To The Pediatrician With You

Your Heart: Questions You Have ... Answers You Need

100 WAYS TO LIVE TO 100

Charles B. Inlander & Marie Hodge

WINGS BOOKS

New York • Avenel, New Jersey

The **People's Medical Society** is a nonprofit consumer health organization dedicated to the principles of better, more responsive and less expensive medical care. Organized in 1983, the People's Medical Society puts previously unavailable medical information into the hands of consumers so that they can make informed decisions about their own health care.

Membership in the People's Medical Society is $20 a year and includes a subscription to the People's Medical Society Newsletter. For information, write to the People's Medical Society, 462 Walnut Street, Allentown, PA 18102, or call (215) 770-1670.

This 1994 edition is published by Wings Books, distributed by Outlet Book Company, Inc., a Random House Company, 40 Engelhard Avenue, Avenel, New Jersey 07001, by arrangement with the People's Medical Society, Inc.

Random House
New York • Toronto • London • Sydney • Auckland

Printed and bound in the United States of America

Library of Congress Cataloging-in-Publication Data
Inlander, Charles B.
  100 ways to live to 100 / Charles B. Inlander and Marie Hodge.
    p. cm.
  Originally published: People's Medical Society, 1992.
  ISBN 0-517-10017-7
  1. Longevity. 2. Aged--Health and hygiene. I. Hodge, Marie.
  II. Title. III. Title: One hundred ways to live to 100.
  RA776. 75. I54   1994
  613' .0438--dc20
                                                    93-43360
                                                    CIP

8 7 6 5 4 3 2 1

Contents

Acknowledgments

All books are collaborative efforts and this one is no exception. The authors wish to thank Jeff Blyskal for practical support above and beyond the call of duty; Krishni Patrick for her cheerful and creative approach to research; Margaret Pierpont for her great ideas and expertise; Tracy Baldwin for her readable and superb designs; Eric Rinehimer for his sharp eye and precision; and Karen Kemmerer for overseeing the production process.

Special thanks to Karla Morales, vice president for communications and editorial services at the People's Medical Society, who served as the executive editor of this book and as overall supervisor of this project. Her tireless efforts and eye for detail are the primary reason an idea became a book. She is greatly appreciated.

The Iowa Department of Elder Affairs deserves particular mention for its unique helpfulness in providing us with persons 100 years of age and older to interview. We are forever grateful for their assistance.

We have tried to use male and female pronouns in an egalitarian manner throughout this book. Any imbalance in usage has been in the interest of readability.

Introduction

I would like to live to be 100. I want to be active, healthy and productive. I want to be happy, have lots of friends and be as independent as possible. I am willing to endure a few setbacks along the way – I recognize that nothing in life is easy. But I want to know what I can do to help my chances of achieving my goal.

To fulfill my quest, several years ago I started looking at the books and articles that had been written about living long. It immediately struck me that none of the great health gurus – individuals who proffered wisdom on living long or staying healthy – had ever lived to be 100. In fact, most had not lived to be even 75, with some notables dying in their 60s or earlier.

I was amazed I could not find a book that carried unbiased information on what a person could do to live long. Most of these tomes were merely one person's recipe for longevity, a formula that usually included buying a product that the author manufactured or going to a spa or clinic he owned.

I turned to the broadcast media. I saw commercial after commercial implying that if I bought the products I might survive longer than the average American. But did I see people who had lived a long life hawking the products? Not once! Either I saw 20-year-old models pumping iron, portly (but no longer obese) former athletes touting diet programs, or over-the-hill movie stars sweating through strenuous exercise. And once again none of them were beyond their 60s. In fact, every time I saw one of these "prophets of health" I would ask myself, "What does he know?"

Like Ponce de Leon, I decided to first search for the secrets to a long life in Florida. My trip wasn't to find the Fountain of Youth, however, but rather to visit my parents, who had retired there a decade before. What I noted in Florida were the huge numbers of people in their 70s, 80s and 90s who were living happy and healthy lives. This scene gave me an idea.

I wrote a short article in the People's Medical Society *Newsletter* asking people who were 70 and older to write and tell me their secrets to longevity. I was overwhelmed with mail. I got letters from men and women ranging in age from 70 to over 100. Everyone had advice for me. I read each letter and later summarized their advice in another People's Medical Society publication.

All the letters were upbeat. These were obviously people who sought to get the most out of life. And by the way, just about every one of them had suffered at least one major health setback at one time or another.

Their letters were truly inspirational. Nobody had lived long by taking magic potions. None wrote that they grew up pampered and overly protected. These were letters from hard-working people who credited their longevity to everything from the food they ate to the genes they inherited—with many more reasons stuffed in between.

I decided to take my search two steps further. First, I thought it was important to go through the medical studies and other scientific literature to find out what experts in particular fields had to tell me about ways to avoid certain diseases and other medical problems. I also wanted to know what the studies told me about additional precautions or actions a person could take that would help ensure longevity.

The second step was to talk to 100-year-old people. If you want to get the inside scoop on anything, always go to the source. In this case, it meant interviewing as many people as possible who had lived at least a century.

For help with both projects I turned to Marie Hodge. Marie is a well-known writer whose career has included many a medical and health journey. She is a senior editor with the magazine *Longevity*, so she quickly understood what we needed to do.

The results are what you will find on the pages that follow. We have looked through the most important medical and scientific studies to provide you with 100 things you can do to improve your chances of living to 100. And we have talked to scores of people 100 years of age or older. The result, I am sure you will agree, is the most useful and inspiring information for living a long life that you have ever found in the pages of one book.

The surprising thing is just how simple most of these tips are. You won't have to go out and buy $500 worth of gymnasium equipment. Nor will you have to order foods with funny-sounding names from countries on the State Department's health-advisory list. You won't even have to buy a juicer, a videotape or a diet pill.

100 Ways to Live to 100 is the best advice from the documented scientific studies and the wisdom of people who have lived a century or more.

Now more than ever I want to live to be 100. Through the research we have conducted and the ideas and knowledge I have learned from people already there, I think making it to 100 is a realistic and exciting goal.

Charles B. Inlander
President
People's Medical Society

1 | Nutrition

The scene is the twenty-second century. A man who was cryo-
genically frozen in 1973 has just been awakened.

Doctor One: Has he asked for anything special?

Doctor Two: Yes, this morning for breakfast. He requested
something called wheat germ, organic honey
and tiger's milk.

Doctor One: Oh yes, those were the charmed substances
that some years ago were felt to contain life-
preserving properties.

Doctor Two: What, no deep fat, no steak or cream pies or
hot fudge?

Doctor One: Those were thought to be unhealthy—
precisely the opposite of what we now know
to be true.
—From Woody Allen's *Sleeper*

Every day there's a new headline hyping the magic health
benefits of yet another food—from oatmeal to tofu to
red wine. But don't worry if you hate oatmeal or tofu—
when it comes to "health" foods, today's hero is likely to be
tomorrow's goat anyway.

As a result, many consumers have the same sneaking
suspicion Woody Allen must have had when he wrote the
above scene for his futuristic film *Sleeper*—that someday the
experts will tell us what our bodies really need is more sugar
and fat after all.

It stands to reason that depending on daily reports from
the research front is not a very good idea. When we hear
about a new study, we can't put it into the context of research
that has gone before or may be going forward simultaneously.
We don't always understand the limits of a particular study's
design or the political pressures on a given researcher as he or
she struggles for grant money. Besides, all nourishment affects
the human body in so many ways—and interacts with other

nourishment in such complex ways – that no one study could give us the total picture.

But take heart; certain broad nutritional truths have hung around long enough to attain solid credibility. Here's what the scientific world knows – or very strongly suspects – about the way you need to eat to live a long life.

1 | If You're Eating the Typical American Diet, It's Time To Reduce Fats and Cholesterol

The single most important step you can take to prolong your life, next to quitting smoking, may be reducing saturated fat and cholesterol in your diet. Study after study has shown that a high-fat diet contributes significantly to heart disease, the number-one killer in America, as well as to a wide variety of common cancers, including those of the breast, colon and ovaries.

Typically, fat makes up about 40 percent of the American diet; all the official government and medical groups say it should be reduced to 30 percent. And of that 30 percent, only one-third should be saturated fat.

But that 30 percent figure is a ceiling, not necessarily an ideal. Privately, some medical experts admit they've reduced their own consumption of fats even more – sometimes to as low as 10 percent. That's because studies have shown fat is a killer.

It's taken many years for public consciousness to catch up to medical discoveries. As long ago as 1911, doctors found evidence that Americans' arteries were being clogged and narrowed by fatty plaque, a process called *atherosclerosis*. In 1955 W.F. Enos Jr., and colleagues, demonstrated evidence of coronary disease in the arteries of 77 percent of the soldiers they studied, men who had been killed in the Korean War and subsequently autopsied. Their average age: 22. Later studies of soldiers killed in Vietnam demonstrated similar results. More recently, a study at Louisiana State University Medical Center found the beginnings of atherosclerosis in the arteries of children as young as six.

In the last few decades, researchers have been steadily investigating the complex ways in which food, heredity, exercise level and other variables interact to clog and narrow arteries to the heart and brain, leading to heart attacks and stroke. So many studies have confirmed the relationship between elevated blood-cholesterol levels and atherosclerosis that there can no longer be any doubt of the connection. Chapter 7 discusses the body's cholesterol level in more detail. Here, we describe how cholesterol level is affected by the foods you choose to eat.

2 | Do Your Math Homework To Determine Fat Content

All right, so nobody likes to do math up and down a super-market aisle. But if you want to stick to the 30 percent ceiling for fat, you've got to do a little each time you go shopping, at least until you become fat-and-cholesterol literate. How do you know how much fat a product contains?

Each gram of fat equals nine calories. A product with five grams of fat would therefore contain 45 calories' worth of fat. If the product is only 100 calories in total, you'd better watch out; 45 of those 100 calories, or 45 percent of calories, are derived from fat.

Unfortunately, you can't simply take the manufacturer's word for fat percentages, because the area is an unregulated land mine. The label on a package of hot dogs or sausage might say "30 percent fat"—but the manufacturer could be measuring the fat content by weight, not by calories. When measured properly, an ordinary package of hot dogs, sausages, bologna or salami would be closer to a whopping 70 or 80 percent fat—giving new meaning to the phrase "lethal weapon."

Of course, any diet can sustain an occasional high-fat jolt if the overall picture is still good. Experts are divided as to whether your 30 percent (or lower) fat average should be measured by the day or by the week, but most people's lives are too complex to keep weekly food diaries. An overall commitment to emphasize low-fat foods, coupled with an informal running tally in your head each day, should be enough for any individual. The longer you pursue this course of action, the more accurate your measurements and estimates become.

G.A., 100, of Ottumwa, Iowa, says taking care of your body is the key to long life. He describes himself as a meat-and-potatoes man who doesn't "eat everything I want to." G.A., a former quality inspector at a nearby food processing plant, sticks to the basic nutrients—fruits, vegetables, grains and meat—and tries to keep his culinary vices, coffee and sugar, in check. He doesn't drink or smoke, doesn't take medicine unless it's necessary and has led a good Christian life both in good times and in bad. "You can't abuse your body; you can't make a garbage can out of it," he stresses.

3 | Do Your Math Homework To Determine Cholesterol Content

Many people think that cholesterol in the blood, or *serum cholesterol,* is affected only by the cholesterol in our diets. While there is a relationship between the two, serum cholesterol is manufactured in the liver and is actually affected more by the saturated fat in our diets than by the cholesterol we eat. Thus, as strange as it may sound, a product labeled "low in cholesterol" can still be bad for your serum cholesterol if it's high in saturated fat.

Nevertheless, dietary cholesterol still has an impact on your cholesterol level and should be reduced to less than 300 milligrams a day, according to the American Heart Association. That's particularly daunting for men, since the average American male consumes about 450 mg. a day (as opposed to 320 mg. for women). Egg yolks and organ meats (liver, sweetbreads, kidney and brain) contain the most cholesterol; a single egg yolk has a cholesterol count of 213 mg.

4 | Make Meat An Accompaniment, Not a Centerpiece

Dietary cholesterol is found only in the animal products we consume, not in the plants, and saturated fat is generally more plentiful in animal products, too. The two greatest sources of saturated fat in our diets are meat and dairy products; the single greatest source of cholesterol is egg yolks (egg whites are mostly protein). In the case of meat, you don't have to give it up completely to live a long life, but you may have to cut back drastically on quantity. Simply going for leaner cuts doesn't necessarily cut it (although whatever cuts you use should be lean; see Table 1-1).

Confusing? The United States Department of Agriculture (USDA) thought so. In early 1992, over the protests of the meat and dairy industries, they revamped the traditional four food groups into five with the "Food Guide Pyramid" (see Figure 1-1). Although the USDA insists the pyramid isn't a ranking of good and bad foods, it clearly recommends many more servings of low-fat foods than of high-fat meats, oils and dairy products.

Table 1-1 | More Healthful Meats

Listed below are cuts of meat that are lean and less mean to your health—lower in saturated fat than other cuts. When choosing grade, remember that higher grades (such as "prime" and "choice") actually contain *more* fat. All three-ounce (cooked) servings of meats should be broiled, roasted or braised, not fried.

Beef	**Pork**
Eye round	Tenderloin
Top round	Extra-lean boneless ham
Tip round	**Veal**
Poultry	Leg
Skinless chicken or turkey breast	Sirloin
Skinless chicken drumstick	
Skinless turkey leg	

Figure 1-1

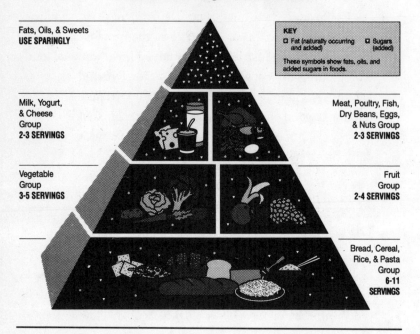

Food Guide Pyramid
A Guide to Daily Food Choices

Fats, Oils, & Sweets
USE SPARINGLY

KEY
▫ Fat (naturally occurring   ▫ Sugars
   and added)   (added)

These symbols show fats, oils, and
added sugars in foods.

Milk, Yogurt,
& Cheese
Group
2-3 SERVINGS

Meat, Poultry, Fish,
Dry Beans, Eggs,
& Nuts Group
2-3 SERVINGS

Vegetable
Group
3-5 SERVINGS

Fruit
Group
2-4 SERVINGS

Bread, Cereal,
Rice, & Pasta
Group
**6-11
SERVINGS**

Fat doesn't just come from butter and sour cream. Ask any American what he's having for dinner, and he may say "hamburgers" or "chicken"—because our culture sees meat as the centerpiece of a meal. The Food Guide Pyramid heralds a new era with a radical new mind-set: Potatoes, pasta, rice, cereal and breads are the true foundation of a good diet, followed closely by vegetables and fruits.

But don't we need lots of meat for protein? Apparently not. Paul Thomas of the Food and Nutrition Board at the National Academy of Sciences says we get protein from many sources, including nuts, beans, peas, dairy products and cereal grains.

In fact, the average American consumes from 1½ to 2 times the amount of protein needed daily, so a serious deficiency is hardly likely. The USDA says we need no more than two or three servings of meat (a serving is three ounces cooked) a day; many Americans get this at one sitting.

5 | ## Choose Low-fat Dairy Products, and Don't Overestimate the Amount You Need

We've all become educated about terms like "2 percent milk" and "skim milk"—or have we? The percentage-of-fat figures that come on milk cartons, like those on packages of hot dogs, are measured by weight, not by calories. If manufacturers were more honest, whole milk would be "50 percent" milk (with 50 percent of its calories derived from fat) and so-called 2 percent milk would be "38 percent" milk. In either case, you clearly don't need the high fat content (unless you're under the age of two; studies have shown that very young children do indeed need the fat of whole milk).

As with meat, many Americans could do with reducing their consumption of dairy products. Even those who have a high calcium requirement—the young and the old—need no more than three one-cup dairy servings a day, which means perhaps milk in morning cereal and coffee (one serving), a glass of milk at lunch, and a low-fat yogurt snack. When you do take in dairy products, go for the leanest versions you can find: low-fat (1 percent) or skim milk, cheeses and yogurts.

Cheese presents a particular problem, because many people see it as a reasonable alternative protein source when they cut back on meat. But many cheeses are very high in saturated fat, sometimes containing as much as ice cream. Your best cheese sources are low-fat cottage cheese, part-skim mozzarella, ricotta and some other softer cheeses.

The American Heart Association recommends you limit eggs to four a week, since egg yolks are high in cholesterol and saturated fat. You can extend your ration of eggs a bit by substituting an egg white for every other whole egg called for in a recipe.

When it comes to long-life prescriptions, Verne Gaskins of Milford, Iowa, is the exception that proves the rule. He has run afoul of all we now know about heart-stopping eating habits and, at age 100, has earned the right to tell the experts they're wrong—at least some of the time! All his life Verne has loved fried foods, bacon and just about anything else nutritionists and doctors consider bad these days. His favorite food: beef. And what about rich fat-filled ice cream? Every night!

Verne's daughter, Jeane Herr, says her father is in another high-risk category: "He's a workaholic!" she exclaims. Verne worked long hours as a pharmacist, and when he wasn't doing that, he'd take on carpentry projects and yard work around the house. "He can't sit still," says Jeane.

So Verne's prescription to those who would follow in his footsteps should not come as a surprise. "When people ask why he's lived so long," explains his daughter, "he replies, 'Hard work and a wife who took care of him and was a good cook.'"

Substitute margarine for butter and lard, but use it sparingly. Margarine is lower in saturated fat than butter but it's high in overall fat. Needless to say, ice cream and cream should be only an occasional treat.

In fact, be careful of all desserts. While the jury is still out on the effects of sugar on long life, there's no question that most desserts are dangerous for high fat content alone. A slice of cake or a scoop of ice cream should be limited to a couple of times a week.

6 | When You Choose Cooking Oils, Emphasize Those With Low Saturated Fat and High Monounsaturated Fat

Fats and oils come in three varieties—saturated, polyunsaturated and monounsaturated. Each of these has a specific effect on serum cholesterol. Saturated oils increase the body's LDL cholesterol (the "bad" kind that contributes to the buildup of fatty plaques in the arteries). The other two kinds, when used in place of saturated fat, actually reduce LDLs. So saturated oils are the most damaging. Does that make the other two equal?

Not quite. While both polyunsaturated and mono- unsaturated reduce LDL, a study at the University of Texas Health Science Center in Dallas showed that polyunsaturates also reduce HDL—the "good" cholesterol that protects against atherosclerosis. That leaves monounsaturated oils the winner and still champ.

Your best bets for cooking are the monounsaturated oils known as canola (rapeseed) and olive oil. The oils to be avoided—those with the most saturated fat—are coconut oil (87 percent) and palm-kernel oil (81 percent). Table 1-2 lists the best and worst oils and fats in terms of their saturated or monounsaturated composition. Don't deep-fry anything, and if you sauté, use as little oil as possible.

Table 1-2 | Saturated vs. Monounsaturated Fats*

Kind of fat	% Saturated	% Monounsaturated
Canola (rapeseed) oil	7	56
Safflower oil	9	12
Sunflower oil	10	20
Corn oil	13	24
Olive oil	14	74
Soft-tub margarine	14	14
Stick margarine	15	37
Peanut oil	17	46
Chicken fat	30	45
Pork lard	40	45
Palm oil	49	37
Beef tallow	50	42
Cocoa butter	60	33
Butter	62	29
Palm-kernel oil	81	11
Coconut oil	87	6

*The numbers on the table do not add up to 100 percent. You should be aware that the difference is accounted for by polyunsaturated fat.

Source: Food and Nutrition Board, Institute of Medicine, National Academy of Sciences.

7 | Eat Fatty Fish Several Times a Week

There is one kind of fat you actually can (and probably should) eat more of—fish fat. Research shows that the more you consume of fish that are high in omega-3 fatty acids, the better your protection from atherosclerosis. In fact, some researchers have found that fish oil lowers blood pressure and even decreases inflammation from arthritis. Of course, recent news stories have cast doubts on the safety of fish, which are easily contaminated by the polluted waters in which they swim. But some kinds of fish are a safer bet than others. (For more information on fish safety, see Chapter 5).

While many kinds of fish are oily enough to contain significant deposits of omega-3 fatty acids, the following fish are particularly high in those fats and should probably be eaten two or three times a week:

- Bluefin tuna
- Herring
- Mackerel
- Salmon
- Shark
- Striped bass
- Turbot (flatfin)

8 | Eat More Grains of A Wider Variety

Our ancestors were right when they dubbed bread the staff of life—we need more daily servings from this food group than from any other. The Food Guide Pyramid recommends from 6 to 11 servings of grains a *day*, depending on your age and gender (children and men need more). Grains are an important source of fiber—the portion of plant foods that humans cannot digest. Fiber has been credited with everything from curing constipation to preventing colon cancer to lowering cholesterol. But fiber comes in two distinct forms, and each has its use.

Of particular help in preventing colon cancer is insoluble fiber, which is found in most bran cereals, whole grains, dried beans and peas (as well as in fruits and vegetables; see below). If your family history includes colon cancer, this is a category you cannot afford to shortchange.

Soluble fiber is equally beneficial, though in a different way. A study by James Anderson, M.D., professor of medicine and clinical nutrition at the University of Kentucky College of Medicine, found that in conjunction with a low-fat, low-cholesterol diet, soluble fiber was effective in lowering cholesterol and triglyceride levels in the blood, both of which are implicated in heart disease. Because it absorbs water in the stomach and intestines, soluble fiber has the extra advantage of making you feel full.

Among the sources of soluble fiber are:
- Carrots
- Corn
- Dried beans
- Lentils

- Oat bran
- Peas
- Prunes

9 | Emphasize Vegetables And Fruits; They're Your First Line of Defense Against Cancer and Heart Disease

Scientists theorize that because humans evolved as vegetarians, our bodies are designed to live longer and work better when we nourish them with the vitamins, minerals and other nutrients most commonly found in vegetables, fruits and grains. Of particular interest to long-life advocates are beta-carotene, which is converted to vitamin A in the body, and vitamins C and E. These three nutrients are called *antioxidants* because they keep destructive forces called free radicals from oxidizing and damaging healthy cells. For that reason, they're thought to be effective in protecting the body from cancer and heart disease. At the same time, they apparently boost the effectiveness of the immune system against all disease.

The carotenoids, of which beta-carotene is the most abundant, help protect the body against cancer. They're most abundant in red, yellow, orange and green vegetables—the deeper the color the higher their level. To get a wide variety of carotenoids into your diet, choose from among different "color groups." Among your 3 to 5 daily servings of vegetables and 2 to 4 servings of fruit (one-half cup each), find a place for some of these high-carotenoid vegetables and fruits:

- Broccoli
- Cantaloupe

- Carrots
- Dried apricots
- Kale
- Pumpkin
- Spinach
- Sweet potato
- Tomatoes
- Winter squash

Other studies have indicated that cruciferous vegetables, those in the cabbage family, contain compounds that break down cancer-promoting chemicals. The cruciferous vegetables include:

- Broccoli
- Brussels sprouts
- Cabbage
- Cauliflower
- Kale
- Rutabaga
- Turnips

Since broccoli and kale are both cruciferous and carotenoid-rich, they should command a prominent place in any long-life diet.

10 | Learn Which Vitamin And Mineral Supplements Are Right for You—and Make Them Part of Your Daily Life

It has taken the medical establishment many years to find out what alternative health practitioners have been saying all along: Vitamins and minerals hold the key to preventing (and maybe even curing) a host of life-shortening ills, from cancer to osteoporosis to heart disease. A growing body of literature in established medical journals indicates that above and beyond our basic vitamin intake from food, most of us could use supplements of some vitamins to extend life and health. It simply isn't possible to get enough of antioxidant vitamins, such as C and E, from a daily diet, however balanced. RDAs (Recommended Daily Allowances) are far behind the times, since they're based on the amount of each vitamin needed to prevent deficiency diseases (such as rickets and scurvy).

Exactly which vitamin and mineral supplements you need depends on your age, sex and physical condition. For example, a recent British study showed that women who take folic acid during the first six weeks of pregnancy are much less likely to give birth to children with neural-tube defects such as spina bifida. Other studies have demonstrated that postmenopausal women need increased calcium to combat loss of bone-mineral density, a condition that results in crippling osteoporosis. Smokers have been advised to increase their intake of vitamin C, and so forth.

Of course, you can't simply consume large doses of selected vitamins indiscriminately. For one thing, too much of one vitamin or mineral might decrease your body's ability to absorb and utilize another. More important, some of the vitamins and minerals so beneficial in small doses are actually toxic in large doses. For example, there is reason to suspect that potassium deficiency might contribute to high blood pressure. But too much potassium can be harmful to the heart if the kidneys don't eliminate it properly, so potassium supplements have to be monitored by a doctor.

If you wish to use supplements as an extra boost to a diet already rich in vitamin-heavy fruits and vegetables, the wisest course is to learn all you can about how vitamins and minerals function in the body—and which supplements are recommended for your particular situation. Two good sources of information are *The Complete Book of Vitamins and Minerals for Health*, by the Editors of *Prevention* Magazine (Emmaus: Rodale, 1988) and *The Vitamin and Mineral Encyclopedia* by Sheldon Saul Hendler (New York: Simon & Schuster, 1990). Armed with information, you can then consult a doctor who is knowledgeable about nutrition and possibly a qualified nutritionist as well. The payoff for taking such good care of your body should be longer life—with a healthier, more vital feel to it.

11 | Get Rid of Excess Salt In Your Diet

For years people with hypertension (high blood pressure)—a significant risk factor in heart disease, stroke and kidney disease—have been told to limit their salt intakes. Salt helps the body retain fluids and pushes high blood pressure up even higher. But do you need to pay attention to your salt intake if your blood pressure is normal?

The answer is, unfortunately, yes. Hypertension specialists believe that some people are more sensitive to the effects of salt than others, but they have no way of knowing who is who until high blood pressure strikes. Someday in the future, a simple test may tell you whether you need to behave as if salt can harm you. But in the meantime, the safest course is to assume that it can. This is particularly important if your family history includes high blood pressure or other cardiovascular problems, diabetes or kidney conditions, or if you're overweight —all risk factors in their own right.

A.B. of Oak Hill, Ohio, is a no-nonsense 103-year-old. When it comes to eating, she does what seems right but has never made a big deal of following prescriptive advice.

"I smoked and drank and did everything ornery," she sniffs. But she has always known how to take care of herself: She takes "a few vitamins every day" but "no other medication," and she uses moisturizing soaps and lotions on her "rather youngish" skin.

A.B. takes pride in being totally self-sufficient and attributes her many years to "being a good person." Her advice to others who want to live to be 100 is to have a strong moral compass. "Behave yourself," she says simply.

Americans typically eat 10 grams of salt a day; that contrasts sharply with the 5 g. of salt (2,000 mg.) the American Heart Association recommends for people with mild or moderate high blood pressure. Giving your saltshaker the heave-ho is a good first step, because 18 percent of the salt in our diets comes to us from the shaker. But if you're going to sharply reduce salt intake, you've got to make an assault on processed foods.

Processed foods tend to have high sodium contents because manufacturers have found salt to be a quick, cheap way to add flavor and extend shelf life at the same time. But the result is that we get 67 percent of our salt this way. Sodium lurks in virtually every canned or frozen good, even some marked "lower in sodium" (since "lower than astronomical" can still be pretty high in its own right).

Salt can be fairly straightforward to measure; if you set yourself a maximum of 2,000 mg. of salt a day and don't use salt at the table, simply tally up the number of milligrams of sodium in your processed goods. Keep a reserve of 15 percent for natural foods and water; that's how much of our salt comes from those sources.

2 | Exercise

Our forebears would have been bewildered at the notion of a formal exercise program; often they toiled in the fields from sunup to sundown, doing back-breaking work that–purely as a side benefit–kept them fit as a fiddle. If they found a spare moment here or there, they would most likely have used that moment for peaceful activities such as reading, sewing or chats by the fireside. Today, it's more likely that work is our sedentary time, and play involves hard-driving physical activity, such as tennis, biking or jogging.

Yet for many of us, play is just as sedentary as work– a situation that puts our health at risk and shortens our lives. A groundbreaking study of Harvard University alumni by Ralph Paffenbarger Jr., M.D., and associates found that those who regularly exercised–through walking, stair climbing or sports play–significantly decreased their chances of dying from cardiovascular or respiratory disorders. Other research has shown that moderate exercise strengthens the heart, helps us lose weight, lowers cholesterol, reduces blood pressure, helps stave off diabetes, fights osteoporosis and gives a boost to our minds and spirits that helps us approach life more positively.

And although the evidence is a bit more tentative, exercise may even help our bodies fight cancer. The same study of Harvard University alumni found that those who burned more than 2,500 calories a week through physical activity were only half as likely to develop colon cancer as sedentary people.

Experts say the biggest stumbling block to keeping people on the right track is the boredom factor–people simply lose interest quickly in whatever program they start. But because there are many different ways to give the body the workout it needs, a sincere convert can always find something that fits the bill. Here are the different factors to keep in mind as you pursue your fitness goal.

12 | Do Something Physical Every Single Day

For the moment, we're not referring to a formal exercise program; recommendations for that come later. What we're talking about is getting in touch with your own body as a tool meant to be used and enjoyed – for gardening, dancing, long contemplative nature walks, sex, even moonlight swims. This part of the fitness prescription does not have a lot of "shoulds" attached. You don't have to do it for a minimum length of time or get your pulse up to a certain count. All you have to do is revel in the physical joy of being.

S.M. of Wilmerding, Pennsylvania, never hesitated to dip into life in all its variety, and it shows. Now 103, he has tried his hand at dozens of different trades throughout his life: shop work, railroad work, hauling ice or coal, even going into business for himself. When he wasn't earning a living, he "liked to dance and be sociable."

The simple pleasures are still the mainstays of his day; he does all his own housework, continues to socialize and takes a walk every day, "weather permitting." How did he handle stress? "When you have trouble, you just work it out," he says. "You don't let it get you down – you just fight it."

If this sounds a little too metaphysical, consider the fact that many people, especially women who grew up before the attitudes of feminism caught on, have never been encouraged to use their bodies in physical, athletic ways. An unused body, like an unused mind, atrophies and becomes more unusable. When you take this neglected instrument into an aerobics class, however noble your intentions, your body reacts as if you're asking it to do something completely foreign. (And indeed, you are.) A fitness program becomes more doable if you simultaneously take time to get comfortable inside your own physical skin.

13 | To Strengthen Your Heart, Do Something Aerobic For 15 to 60 Minutes a Day, 3 to 5 Times a Week

There's a whole mystique to aerobic movement, and some of it is unnecessary – it isn't an impenetrable mystery. Aerobic exercise simply involves any whole-body, rhythmic, repetitive activity that makes your heart beat faster and your breath come a little harder – period. It can be running, dancing, swimming, bicycling, skating, fast walking, even jumping on a pogo stick.

How fast do you need to exercise to give your heart an aerobic workout? It's less intense than you might think. There are two ways to measure your output: one is purely subjective, the other a more objective measurement – pulse rate. Some people become impatient measuring pulse; others find it a reassuring double check. Your choice should be the approach that best fits your personality and temperament.

The subjective measurement is known as "perceived exertion," and studies show that it correlates well with more objective measures. Simply put, it means that you should walk or dance or swim or whatever at a pace brisk enough to make you feel it's kind of hard – but not too hard. If your breath is coming in great gasps and sweat is pouring down your face, you've gone too far. On the other hand, if your breathing has hardly changed at all, you haven't gone far enough. For many people, that's all they need to know to determine whether their bodies are getting aerobic benefits.

For a more objective measurement, follow the American College of Sports Medicine (ACSM) guidelines for pulse rate, based on age. The ACSM says your workout should be at 60 to 90 percent of your maximum heart rate (the rate your heart pumps when it's working as hard as it possibly can). If you've had a stress test, you probably know what that is. If not, the general rule of thumb is to start from the number 220 and subtract your age. So if you're 40, your maximum heart rate is 180. You do not have to exercise at the maximum to get aerobic benefits.

In this example, the lowest *target* heart rate – the one you're shooting for when you exercise aerobically – would be 108 (60 percent of 180), the highest would be 162 (90 percent of 180). If you've led a sedentary life for years, it may be wisest to start at the lowest number in the target range and work your way up. On the other hand, if your job involves hard physical labor or you engage regularly in fitness-building sports, you may be able to start at a higher target heart rate. Gear your approach to your needs as an individual, and don't forget to see a doctor first.

14 | Build Up Your Muscles And Bones

Aerobic benefit is one thing, but if you want long life with maximum health, you have to build up your muscles and bones. As your body ages, it has a tendency to put on weight; if you're not making it into muscle, it will probably become fat. Muscle cells also help keep weight down because they burn more calories than fat cells do.

In addition, putting some stress on muscles helps combat loss of bone density, an ongoing process that begins when women are still in their 30s (and can sometimes affect men later in life). Loss of density gradually results in *osteoporosis*, the disease that makes women's bones brittle and easily broken as they grow older. Those easily broken bones—particularly in the hip and the pelvis—put women into the hospital and often lead to a debilitating downward spiral in health.

Studies at Tufts University's USDA Human Nutrition Research Center on Aging show that the natural muscle loss that accompanies aging can be reversed with weight-bearing exercises. For these purposes, split the body into two halves—the upper and lower body. If you're already doing aerobic exercise that places weight on your lower body (running or walking, for example), you've probably begun to build muscles in that area. If so, you should concentrate on building muscles and strengthening bones in the upper body.

Muscle building can be accomplished in a number of ways. The most straightforward is to go to a well-equipped fitness center—which may be no more exotic than your local YMCA—and ask for a muscle-building program using free weights or machines. Different equipment concentrates on different major muscle groups. Among the 8 to 10 major muscle groups you should be working on are the abdomen, the front thighs, the back thighs, the calves, your hips and buttocks, the chest, the back, and shoulders and arms.

If a fitness center is not your style, or you can't spare the expense, you can follow the basic principles of muscle building in more down-to-earth ways. Using weights is probably the fastest way to get results, but long before the invention of weight-training rooms, people built muscles through exercises like push-ups, squats and knee-bends. For a program geared to your own needs, consult your physician first and then a qualified fitness consultant. Because of the possibility of injury when exercises are not done properly, it isn't advisable to develop your own program without help from an expert.

Incidentally, to protect your muscles, any exercise should begin and end with a less-intense period of five minutes during which the muscles gradually warm up or cool down.

15 | Strengthen Your Abdomen To Help Support Your Back

Much as we may hate to admit it, human beings were originally designed to walk on all fours; standing upright places tremendous strain on our backs. For that reason, back problems are epidemic, and they become more prevalent as we age. Lower-back pain has severe implications for the quality of life; people who suffer from it are more likely to shun exercise and to approach life less positively. The end result may be a body unequipped to tackle the challenge of long life. Beyond weight-bearing exercises (discussed previously) that are designed specifically for the back, the best gift you can give your back is a strong abdomen. Strong abdominal muscles help support the back and keep it from sagging. So when you're strengthening major muscle groups, pay particular attention to your abdomen.

Claire Willi, 102, was born and grew up in the Swiss mountains and emigrated to the United States as a young woman. She's lived a life of grace and elegance. Married for 54 years to a broker who was "the biggest champagne dealer in New York," she once kept up homes in three states.

If you ask Claire what keeps her young, she doesn't beat around the bush: "Exercise," she says. "All my friends are dead because they didn't exercise." At 101 years of age, she was in such good shape that she was able to bound out of a pothole that she had accidentally fallen into.

But Claire wasn't always so spry. At 70, she found herself a "tired, old, run-down woman with feet that hurt all the time." Enter Milton Feher, a former Broadway hoofer whose dance studio helped her get back in shape. Now she goes every single day, and Milton calls her "one of my best dancers . . . very graceful." Claire's advice to longevity seekers: "Stand straight. It's very important."

16 | Keep Your Joints Flexible

If you don't use your joints, quite simply, they'll tighten with age. One day when you go to reach for a high shelf, you'll feel a sudden sharp stab of pain and you'll suffer an injury. Tightened joints also help to create the stooped, shuffling appearance we tend to associate with old age – a definite stumbling block to graceful aging. In addition, studies have shown that people with arthritis experience much less pain if they continue to keep their joints flexible. The basic message is simple: "Use it or lose it."

In recent years, water exercises have become a popular way to exercise and strengthen joints without injuring them. That's because water provides cushioning protection for joints as well as resistance against which to exercise. The latest variation on this is water running, where the runner wears a flotation device to keep afloat, then stands in a pool or other still water and pumps arms and legs to mimic the movement of running on land.

17 | Don't Exercise Just On Weekends

With spare time more plentiful on weekends, many people opt to do the bulk of their exercising then. But this is a mistake, from the points of view of both injury prevention and biochemical benefit. Weekend athletes are exercising muscles and joints that have been lying fallow all week, and it's easier to overtax a muscle or joint in this situation.

More important from the standpoint of long life, researchers at the National Institute on Aging say that all exercise increases the production of free radicals—metabolic by-products that rampage through the body, damaging tissues and contributing to the aging process. If you're exercising regularly, your body is also producing antioxidants to neutralize these free radicals. But if your exercise program is sporadic, your body is not protected by a high-level dose of antioxidants (unless these are part of your personal vitamin-supplement plan; see Chapter 1). Your best bet is to keep to a steady program distributed as evenly as possible throughout the week.

18 | Find an Exercise Program You Love—and Don't Hesitate to Change It

Some 50 percent of people who take up an exercise program stick with it for less than six months. Typically, such people find the routines boring, time consuming and unrewarding. Often they don't "hang in there" long enough to get the thrill of feeling fit—a thrill that keeps many exercise fans coming back.

That's why an important attribute of any successful exercise program is that you love the activity itself. If you can't think of any physical activity you love, go back to your childhood. Did you spend hours roller skating or skipping rope or swimming? Did you often long for a trampoline because it looked like fun? Alternatively, you can take up a new physical activity that looks like it might be fun. If it also happens to be one that your friends, spouse or children like, so much the better; the buddy system is more likely to keep you involved than going solo would. Getting back to the playful feelings inspired by youthful physical activities can help you to enjoy exercise – and stick with it.

At the same time, don't become so wedded to one activity that its novelty value begins to wear off and it starts to feel like work. Experts suggest changing activities often – even within the same workout – to exercise as many different parts of the body as possible and to keep your interest level high. Don't hesitate to go from fast walking to swimming or dancing; you have nothing to lose but your boredom.

19 | Combine Exercise With Stress-Relief Techniques

People who exercise regularly report that they are generally happier and in a more upbeat mood when they have had a workout. There's a biochemical explanation for this: Exercise releases opiatelike substances in the brain called *endorphins,* which improve our mood, make us more optimistic and generally add to the quality of life. While you may find the early stages of a new exercise program somewhat stressful, it's a safe bet that once you're exercising regularly the level of life-shortening stress in your life decreases, thanks to increased endorphin levels.

Unfortunately, the full benefit of endorphins – the so-called exercise high – isn't usually felt until about an hour after you finish a workout. For many people, particularly those in the early stages of a program, a more immediate payoff would give more of an incentive to keep exercising. According to a study by sports psychologist Youde Wang, Ph.D., at the University of Massachusetts Medical Center, people who engage in relaxation techniques while walking show a significantly reduced level of anxiety after each workout than those who simply walk.

What Wang suspects is that many of us ruminate about daily worries or engage in other negative thoughts while we exercise–adding to the stress of the workout. His study subjects listened to relaxation tapes describing breathing and counting techniques designed to focus the mind on something more neutral. But he says simply counting steps or repeating a phrase in your head (a kind of mantra) would work just as well. Either way, to stop your mind from "playing" a tape of negative thoughts while you exercise, train it to focus on something more neutral.

20 | Don't Overlook Opportunities For Exercise in Your Own Backyard

Fitness enthusiasts tend to emphasize certain kinds of athletic physical activities–running, cycling, swimming and others. But if you've never been the athletic type and aren't about to start now, don't despair. Unless you're comatose by nature, you are probably engaging in activities (at least some of the time) that can help you stay fit. Studies show that playing three games of golf a week can drive down your cholesterol if you walk instead of ride a golf cart. Ballroom dancing has been shown to be a fine aerobic workout. And most amazingly of all, you can burn almost as many calories doing housework or gardening as you can with many of the more athletic workouts.

Sound incredible? Just check out the numbers in Table 2-1. A 130-pound woman would use up more calories scrubbing floors for an hour than she would biking during that time. And a 180-pound man would use up more calories chopping wood than he would weight training. The difference is, performing a job around the house offers a payoff of a necessary task being performed—another good exercise incentive.

Table 2-1 | Exercise Is Where You Find It

The following activities vary widely in their ability to burn calories. But it's clear that you don't have to be an Olympic-caliber athlete to give your body a workout.

Activity	Calories Burned (per hour)	
	180-lb. man	130-lb. woman
Ballroom dancing	288	208
Chopping wood	450	350
Cooking	234	162
Cycling	486	351
Gardening	300	220
Jogging	756	546
Jumping rope	684	494
Ironing	312	114
Mowing lawn by hand	320	250
Scrubbing floors	522	377
Skating	468	338
Swimming	630	455
Vacuuming	222	162
Weight training	342	247

21 | Keep an Exercise Diary

A log of your daily physical activities is a good way to reassure yourself of progress being made. Keep track of your resting pulse, exercise pulse, the activity involved, the distance covered, the amount of time involved and the amount of resistance (for weight-training activities). If you begin to find your resting pulse rate going down after a time, that's a good sign; it means your cardiovascular system is beginning to operate with less strain on your body. If you find your times decreasing, it means your body is getting more fit.

You might even keep track of reductions in weight as you exercise. Taking pride in your accomplishments may spur you to continue or even add to your exercise commitment.

22 | If You Want to Decrease One Element of Your Exercise Program, Offset It With An Increase in Another Element

Every exercise program involves at least three elements: distance, intensity and frequency. Any change in one element should be offset by a compensatory change in another. Thus if you can jog only three times in one week instead of your usual four (*frequency*), you might compensate by jogging a greater *distance* or moving at a faster pace (*intensity*). This gives the body a way of keeping on an even keel even when schedules don't. Keep in mind, however, that you can only crank up intensity volume so far before you risk hurting yourself. So your best bet wherever possible is to keep all three elements as consistent as possible.

> **B**ertha Jones, of Woodward, Iowa, has always said hard work, no smoking and no drinking are what have kept her alive for 103 years. As a farm wife, she cultivated a large garden, took care of the farm stock, butchered meat, canned vegetables and fruits and tended to a hundred other chores around the homestead. That hard work may have helped offset her penchant for pork, creamery products and the like—concentrated sources of energy when the body has plenty of good uses for those calories.
>
> Throughout her life, Bertha's good health has kept her in the best location for long life—far away from the doctor's office. And she never let stress or anger attack her system. Her elixir for that: Whenever problems arose, Bertha would remember, "Through faith, we can handle anything."

3 | Heredity

n early 1992, the nation's computer owners were given fair warning. On March 6 – the birth date of Renaissance painter and sculptor Michelangelo – a computer virus would set out to kill the hard-drive memories of personal computers. The so-called Michelangelo virus would stalk only one particular computer type, IBM compatibles, and electronic death would strike only on a specific date. Most important, the infected victims-to-be exhibited certain identifiable traits that gave their owners an early clue to their susceptibility. Armed with this information, owners could follow a program designed to rid their computers of the virus before it could strike.

As things turned out, Michelangelo wasn't much of an epidemic. But within targeted computers' silicon chips there is a lesson about what it takes to survive a full century. All of us carry hereditary traits that put us at higher risk for certain ailments and causes of death. If only we could punch a code into a computer keyboard to reveal the danger signs and focus attention on ridding our bodies of these biological time bombs.

In fact, the information is knowable, but it's hidden in the complex chemistry of our genes. The Human Genome Project, a massive cooperative research undertaking of 3,000 scientists funded by the federal government, is mapping the human body's 100,000+ genes, hoping to crack that code by the year 2004 and identify problem genes that predispose some people to cancers, heart disease or other life-threatening afflictions. That should lead to testing, earlier-than-early detection and prevention. In this futuristic model, people will be tested at birth for susceptibility to diseases that may not strike for 50 or 60 years; that knowledge can provide the power of prevention.

Luckily, we don't have to wait for Buck Rogers to decipher the code; indeed, in the business of preventive medicine, right now is always the best time to start gathering knowledge and taking precautions.

If actress Gilda Radner had explored her family medical

history, she might have beaten her fatal ovarian cancer. Unknown to her, her grandmother, aunt and a cousin had all suffered the same disease. That increased her chances of getting ovarian cancer from just 1.4 percent to 50 percent, which should have helped her be more vigilant. Knowledge is power in beating cancer: The survival rate for ovarian cancer is 85 percent when it's detected early; when it's detected late, the odds for survival plummet to just 15 to 20 percent. For Radner, detection came too late.

By learning your family medical history, you get revealing advance warning about your potential medical destiny. Indeed, your family medical history is a window onto the goings-on at the invisible, molecular, gene level.

Each day, researchers establish more links between disease and genetics. Among the significant conditions that tend to run in families: allergies, alcoholism, Alzheimer's disease, asthma, breast cancer, colorectal cancer, diabetes, heart disease, Huntington's chorea, lung cancer and ovarian cancer.

Here's how to find this life-stretching information and what to do with it.

23 | Make Your Own Medical History to Help Your Doctor Monitor Your Health

If everything worked the way it should, doctors would keep an exhaustive medical history that spanned your entire life and every conceivable condition or physical problem that had affected you or your blood relatives. Most responsible doctors attempt to do something vaguely like this when you first sign on as a patient, but there are limitations on both the doctor's time and your knowledge or memory. If your doctor does not have a category for a specific condition, and your long-ago bout with that condition is not at the forefront of memory, it simply doesn't get reported.

Why does it matter? Because each of the medical events in your life is like a piece of a giant puzzle. For example, even if she hasn't suffered an episode in years, a woman who spent significant portions of her childhood fighting off bronchitis or pneumonia is likely to have a respiratory system susceptible to infection and other problems. She may be more prone to allergy and asthma (a lot of what was called bronchitis in her childhood might today be called asthma). When she goes to her doctor with a "cold," the medication she requires and the care with which the condition is followed up may all be affected by the doctor's knowledge of her previous history.

Experts say the inability to make a conclusive diagnosis is one of the weakest links in modern medicine. If this woman and her doctor were both aware of her history, it would help in early diagnosis and effective treatment—two of the most important disease fighters we have. To help jog your memory and to help your doctor compile a full and accurate record of your all-important medical history, fill out Table 3-1. Take it with you when you visit your doctor.

Table 3-1 | Condition Profile Checklist

THIS RECORD BELONGS TO: _____

Date of Birth _____ Place of Birth _____

Insurance Company _____

ID# _____ Telephone _____

Medicare Number _____

Indicate by check mark those conditions which you have/had.

BLOOD

___ Bleeding tendency

___ Bruise easily

___ Hemolytic anemia

___ Other anemia

BONES, MUSCLES & JOINTS

___ Arthritis

___ Backache

___ Bone tumors

___ Fractures

___ Muscle Pain

___ Osteomyelitis

DIGESTIVE – STOMACH & INTESTINE

___ Appetite changes

___ Blood-streaked stools

___ Diverticulitis

___ Gallbladder disease

___ Hemorrhoids

___ Tarry Stools

___ Tumors – stomach, colon, rectum

___ Ulcers

___ Weight gain

___ Weight loss

EARS

___ Deafness

___ Dizziness

___ Drainage from ears

___ Hearing aid

___ Ringing in ears

EYE

___ Blurred vision

___ Cataracts

___ Double vision

___ Eye infection

___ Glaucoma

___ Sudden blindness

GENITAL & URINARY

___ Bloody urination

___ Excessive urination

___ Kidney stones

___ Losing urine when coughing, straining, laughing, etc.

___ Painful urination

___ Urinary-tract infections

___ Urination at night

(continued)

Table 3-1 | Condition Profile Checklist (*continued*)

GLANDS & HORMONES

___ Diabetes

___ Goiter (enlarged thyroid)

___ Persistent fever

___ Protruding eyeballs

___ Sugar in urine

___ Thyroid tumors

___ Unusual thirst

___ Weakness and general tiredness

HEART & LUNGS

___ Abnormal electrocardiogram

___ Ankle and leg swelling

___ Asthma

___ Blueness of lips and fingers

___ Bronchitis

___ Chest pain

___ Chest x-ray abnormalities

___ Chronic cough

___ Coughing up blood

___ Fainting with coughing

___ Heart attack

___ Heart enlargement

___ Heart murmur

___ High blood pressure

___ Irregular heartbeats

___ Leg cramps

___ Low blood pressure

___ Lung tumors

___ Night sweats

___ Pneumonia

___ Shortness of breath at night

___ Shortness of breath lying down

___ Shortness of breath upon exertion

___ TB or TB exposure (tuberculosis)

___ Thrombophlebitis

___ Varicose veins

INFECTIOUS DISEASES

___ Chicken pox (varicella)

___ German measles (rubella)

___ Gonorrhea

___ Measles (rubeola)

___ Mumps (parotitis)

___ Syphilis

MALES

___ Difficulty starting stream

___ Prostate tumor

___ Sexual dissatisfaction

___ Sexual impotency

___ Sore on penis

___ Urethral infection

NERVE DISORDERS

___ Convulsive disorder

___ Difficulty with limb control

___ Extremities fall "asleep"

___ Head trauma

___ Headache

___ Memory problem

___ Muscle weakness

___ Speech problem

___ Stroke

___ Tremor (shaking)

___ Walking disorder

NOSE

___ Deviated septum

___ Nosebleeds

___ Polyps

___ Runny nose

___ Sinusitis

OBSTETRICS & GYNECOLOGY

___ Abnormal Pap smear

___ Abnormal breast exam

___ Abnormal pelvic exam

___ Age began menstruating

___ Bleeding between periods

___ Menopause

___ Miscarriages

___ Painful intercourse

___ Painful menstruation

___ Post-menopause bleeding

___ Pregnancy

___ Sexual dissatisfaction

___ Tumors – breast, uterus, cervix, ovaries, etc.

___ Vaginal infections

SKIN

___ Changes in wart, mole, etc.

___ Chronic skin infections/lesions

___ Common skin infections

___ Psoriasis

___ Skin rash

___ Skin sensitive to light

___ Skin tumors

(continued)

Table 3-1 | Condition Profile Checklist (*continued*)

THROAT

___ Difficulty swallowing   ___ Recurrent sore throat

___ Mouth infections   ___ Sore tongue

___ Persistent hoarseness   ___ Voice change

FAMILY MEDICAL HISTORY	Father	Mother	Brothers/Sisters		
Accident	___	___	___	___	___
Alcoholism	___	___	___	___	___
Allergies	___	___	___	___	___
Anemia	___	___	___	___	___
Cancer	___	___	___	___	___
Diabetes	___	___	___	___	___
Headaches	___	___	___	___	___
Hearing Loss	___	___	___	___	___
Heart Attack	___	___	___	___	___
Hypertension	___	___	___	___	___
Kidney	___	___	___	___	___
Obesity	___	___	___	___	___
Psychosis	___	___	___	___	___
Rheumatoid Arthritis	___	___	___	___	___
Stroke	___	___	___	___	___
Tuberculosis	___	___	___	___	___
Age Died	___	___	___	___	___
Cause of Death	___	___	___	___	___

We gratefully acknowledge Woodbridge Press for permitting us to extract material from *Keeping Track: A Personal Health Record System* (Santa Barbara, CA: Woodbridge Press, 1980).

---

24 | To Aid in Early Detection And Treatment of Life-Threatening Conditions, Learn About the Medical Histories of Your Blood Relatives

If your relatives have a significant history of bouts with heart disease, diabetes, osteoporosis or a particular form of cancer, the time to learn about it is now. Armed with that information, you can alter your lifestyle to emphasize prevention strategies, pay close attention to the recommended ages for screening tests, and in some cases, get screened at an earlier age.

The best way to dig out your family medical history is to extract it from living relatives. Make believe you're Phil Donahue and interview relatives about their medical pasts. But be sensitive to the fact that you may be treading on difficult personal ground. For example, older relatives may have grown up believing that there was something shameful about getting cancer—almost as if it were contagious—and may use euphemisms like "he just wasted away." Ask them to tell you what information they'd like you to handle discreetly. Impress upon them the importance of your work and how it could benefit their descendants for generations to come.

Probe for more specifics, but don't press anyone beyond his level of comfort. Another relative may be able to confirm or deny your suspicions about the unspoken diagnosis. If not, compile a list of as many specific symptoms as you can, and measure those symptoms against those found in a good medical guide. Your diagnosis may be tentative, but it's better than none at all.

Your investigation need not be like a military operation to seek and seize information. Collect your data at family gatherings and in casual telephone conversations. Even though your information gathering is relaxed, organization is key. Arrange your information by person and keep all raw data about each person in one place. Each family member should have her own file.

The first files (after your own) should be about your spouse and children. List everything you know about your medical history. From here, move on to your family of origin (and your spouse's), including parents and siblings. These are your first-degree relatives, whose gene makeup is highly similar to yours. Your parents are also a primary source of information about your second-degree relatives—aunts, uncles, grandparents, first cousins. Although they are not as similar genetically to you as first-degree relatives are, start files on them, too. You're looking for patterns that repeat themselves over and over through the generations.

What kind of information are you looking for?

• Vital statistics—birth date, height, weight, occupation, marital status and children

• Medical statistics—cholesterol levels, blood pressure, allergies

• Major and chronic afflictions—everything from heavy-duty cancer and organ diseases to chronic conditions like migraines and asthma

• Details of dead relatives—immediate and underlying causes of death, age at death and where died

• Observations and information about mental health, including depression, anxiety, social withdrawal, explosive behavior, hyperactivity or other problems

• Lifestyle and habits, including diet, exercise, favorite pastimes, consumption of alcohol, tobacco and other drugs

• How stress physically manifested itself in the body—whether through clenched stomach, back pain, headache, fainting or other ways

•Economic, educational and social status. You don't need to see tax forms, but you should get a general idea of your relatives' station, because it can have a great impact on the kinds of health problems they've been exposed to.

Your oral research should extend to your extended family, too. Aunts, uncles and cousins can tell you things your parents don't know; and they might tell you things no one else wants you to know. The more people you talk to, the wider your net is cast to pick up valuable information.

Like many centenarians, Flossie Herwehe, of Norwich, Iowa, hasn't given much thought to why she's lived to age 100. But it is clear that she was blessed with a strong body. Through her long life, she's gone through seven major operations with no ill effects, and not even a fall on the ice in 1971—at age 79—kept her down for good. Flossie comes from a strong bloodline, too: "Dad died when he was only 75," she explains, "but Mom lived to 88."

She respected her body and self, as well. "When I was in school, it got around that I was a good girl. Other girls were loose, but I was never that way," she says. As soon as she graduated from college with a degree in accounting, she married her boyfriend. It should be no wonder, then, that Flossie advises others to "stay on the straight and narrow. Live normally and be good to people."

As a former farm girl, she also recommends a good balanced diet, including plenty of fruits and vegetables. "But I never went overboard," she says. "I don't live to eat, I eat to live."

Grandparents can extend the record of knowledge back further still, because in their day, verbal record keeping was more common. They may know facts that date back several generations. Most important, try to get these basic vital statistics about dead relatives:

- What were their names, including middle initials, nicknames, maiden names, and "Old World" pre-Americanized names?
- Who was related/married/born to whom?
- What were their occupations and places of residence?
- What year did they die?
- Where are they buried?
- What were the causes of death?
- How old were they when they died?
- What city, county and state did they die in?

25 | Examine Written Records Of Your Relatives' Medical Histories—And Add Your Findings to Your Own Medical Record

Grilling your elders about the basics lays the groundwork for another source of information about your family medical history—the documentary record. Like the oral history you've gathered from living relatives, this can help you decide which illnesses you are most at risk for—and how to prevent them.

The primary document you want is the death certificate. It should explain the immediate cause of death and—if there is one—the underlying cause. For example, an automobile accident may have been the immediate cause of death, but a heart attack or stroke could have caused the accident. Pneumonia could have caused the death of a relative, too, but that condition may have been fatal only after a long bout with cancer. Make note of the section "Other Significant Conditions." Age and other vital statistics of the deceased may be useful, too.

Obtain death certificates through your state office of vital statistics, located in the capital. Call that office for information on how to obtain these records. Generally, you need to provide the full name of the deceased, when and where he died (that's why it's vital to get dates from relatives), and your name and relation to the departed. The office of vital statistics may be able to conduct a search for you if your information is vague, but this capability varies from state to state.

Other documentary records are worth obtaining. Marriage certificates (also available from vital-statistics bureaus) can help trace a bride's roots. If your family has an heirloom Bible, it may contain an abundance of information about births, deaths, marriages and significant life events in the family.

A family photo album may also provide useful information. Note weight and build. A *consistent pattern* of facial expressions and attitudes by the same person over time can reveal clues about mental health and general happiness—as with the person who always seems to have a pained smile, a scowl or a pleasant visage. How do the family members in each picture relate to each other? Do they all seem comfortable with each other, or is one person always off to the side or out of sync with the rest of the crowd? Don't expect a full psychological profile from this photo psychoanalysis session, but you can get telling impressions about your kin, and sometimes some solid evidence of medical conditions.

For example, medical experts say photographs of Abraham Lincoln suggest he had symptoms of Marfan's syndrome, a hereditary, degenerative, neurological disorder that would have taken the sixteenth president's life if assassin John Wilkes Booth had not. Similarly, a photography subject's bulging eyes can reveal characteristics of hyperthyroidism – a potentially fatal disease if left untreated.

26 | Make Conclusions About Your Areas of Genetic Vulnerability

By itself, each piece of information gathered in your research tells little about the potential health risks you face. A useful, potentially life-extending picture emerges only when you fit the puzzle pieces together.

For example, if an uncle and one of your parents died of lung cancer and a sister has now developed the disease, you and your clan may be particularly susceptible to that disorder. However, if you have another piece of information – showing that all the victims were smokers – your risk may be less if you are a nonsmoker. (If you are a smoker, however, this is a pretty conclusive indicator that you must stop before you too succumb to the "family weakness.")

Does heart disease or early-age heart attack "run" in your family? If it does, your family may have a genetic predisposition for high cholesterol or simply a weak ticker. But if you link the heart deaths with photos of rotund relatives and evidence of a familial diet high in fat and cholesterol, a change from that family lifestyle can no doubt keep you living longer than your unfortunate relatives.

Above all, avoid becoming superstitious or hypochondriacal. If your grandfather, father and brother died of suicide, there is not necessarily a death warrant on you. However, underlying, unrecognized mental-health problems, like depression, may pass from generation to generation; if you are experiencing any of the symptoms (see Chapter 8), you should err on the side of caution and go to a professional for evaluation.

27 | Alter Your Lifestyle To Prevent the Diseases To Which You're Genetically Susceptible—And Set Up A Plan for Periodic Screenings

Just knowing about the conditions you're at risk for subtly alters your lifestyle in many ways. If you're a good candidate for stroke, and unless you have a death wish, you automatically start paying more attention to cholesterol levels, diet and news about research findings concerning that problem. But this base of knowledge is also power; with it, you can take a more proactive approach to protecting your life and health.

Once you have a bead on the diseases you may be prone to, you can develop a strategy to combat the potential killers in the earliest stages of their development.

The plan involves red-flagging those high-possibility health problems and subjecting them to a periodic schedule of appropriate screening. This involves both objective testing and subjective self-assessment of what your body may be telling you.

Suppose you have found that leukemia runs in your family. So you want to keep an eye out for symptoms of the disease in you and your family—among them, fatigue and other symptoms of anemia, pressure under the left side of your ribs resulting from an enlarged spleen, swollen lymph nodes and weight loss. A good medical guide can provide essential data on symptoms.

But sometimes, there are no overt symptoms, so more-scientific methods may be worth pursuing.

The simplest screen for leukemia is a blood test, including a complete blood count. Indeed, leukemia is often discovered in routine blood testing for other problems before symptoms of this blood cancer present themselves. If chronic myelogenous leukemia (CML) is part of your family tree, you should have your genes screened for the so-called Philadelphia chromosome, which is found in 90 percent of people with CML.

Regular blood testing may be advisable for your young children if your family has a history of acute lymphocytic leukemia (ALL). When detected early in younger children, ALL is successfully treated 70 percent of the time; for older children and adults, the survival rate is only 20 percent.

Other kinds of screening are appropriate for different afflictions—digital rectal exams for prostate cancer, blood pressure and cholesterol tests for heart disease and stroke, mammograms for breast cancer.

Table 3-2 spells out the screening tests you may want to consider if the listed major condition is common to your family.

Rootedness and pioneer endurance seem to be the keys to Ruth Scott's 100 years. Her grandmother Elizabeth, who came to Farragut, Iowa, from Indiana by covered wagon, lived into her 90s. Ruth lived in the same house most of her life. During the depression, however, Ruth struck out for Nebraska with her new husband and endured the dust-bowl days before returning to Farragut.

Most of all, Ruth thanks her genetic strength. "I've never had any serious illness," she says.

28 | If You Have a Strong Family History of Cancer, Consider the Tumor-Marker Blood Test

A new and simpler weapon in the early-detection arsenal is emerging for cancers – tumor-marker blood tests. These tests seek out minuscule amounts of material known to be thrown off into the blood by cancerous tissue. For example, a cancerous ovary secretes a protein known as CA 125, which can be detected with the CA 125 blood test. A colon infected with cancer releases carcinoembryonic antigen into the blood, which can be found with the CEA blood test.

Genetic early-warning tests are also being developed, which can, for example, detect lung cancer based on chromosome abnormalities found in sputum. The Massachusetts Institute of Technology's Arteriosclerosis Center in Boston is even working on a new x-ray test that gives doctors a body-wide picture of exactly where your arteries are constricted and clogged. That kind of noninvasive early detection may mean the problem can be treated with exercise, diet and cholesterol-lowering drugs.

29 | Take Tests With a Grain of Salt

Screening tests – from Pap smears to cholesterol counts – can help add years to your life. But beware, they can also cut your life short and drain your wallet if a test is inaccurate. All screening tests, especially the newest ones, are prone to error—both positive and negative results that are ultimately proven false (known as *false positive* and *false negative*). The new PSA blood test, which plumbs the blood for prostate specific antigens related to prostate cancer, comes up false positive or false negative 36 percent of the time; but the Pap smear produces a false result 35 percent of the time it's positive, too. Even a basic blood-pressure reading can be thrown off if the person administering the test is inexperienced or the cuff is not the right size for the dimensions of a particular arm. A recently developed test is likely to be more prone to error just because the test-givers' body of experience with the test is short-lived and not extensive.

How can testing kill? In most cases a test itself doesn't do that, but an erroneously recommended procedure might. For example, medical experts estimate that 15 to 25 percent of all surgery is unnecessary. Misdiagnosis and/or poor testing creates the justification and demand for that unnecessary surgery. All major surgery involves approximately a 1.3 percent risk of death through complications. A bad test result could send you needlessly into the operating room and on to your grave.

Relatively less dramatic damage can be caused by inaccurate test results: unnecessary removal of an organ, unnecessary chemotherapy or radiation treatment, nonfatal complications, pain or discomfort from a recommended procedure. And all of it invariably leads to a pocketbook "cash-ectomy."

So whenever you are screened, use *all* test results the way the Pentagon uses the Distant Early Warning antinuclear-attack system. When a worrisome blip shows up on their screens, they don't automatically press the button and launch Armageddon; the blip could have been a flock of geese, not incoming nuclear warheads. So, too, when health screens indicate potential trouble for you, don't assume Judgment Day has arrived. Always request reconnaissance – additional or repeat testing, second opinions – to get more evidence to substantiate the early warning.

Because testing can be expensive, consult with your physician to get a professional and gut-level opinion about the need for further testing, factor in cost when choosing tests, and use your own common sense. If three successive tests have found no evidence of the suspected disease but your doctor suggests an $800 magnetic resonance imaging to "eliminate the last 1/10 percent chance," you may want to call off the diagnostic hounds and bet with the odds that are already in your favor.

Ben and Gladys Pruitt, aged 103 and 102, respectively, credit strong genes for their long lives. Ben's oldest sister is also older than 100, and many other family members are in their 90s. Gladys' family members lived mainly into their 80s. Neither has ever smoked, and both shun alcohol and coffee. In fact, they say, none of their long-lived relatives drank coffee.

Gladys also credits an active lifestyle and broad range of interests for their many years. Among their interests: painting, hunting Indian artifacts and studying/hunting mushrooms. Ben has become a recognized authority on mushrooms in his spare time.

Ben and Gladys are living proof that cancer can be beaten. Both had surgery for the disease in 1981 and have fully recovered since. So, they say, they owe a lot to the excellent care they got from their doctors.

Table 3-2 | Nipping Family Diseases in the Bud

If a certain disease or condition runs in your family, you may want to consider the associated screening tests listed below. They can help detect the disease as early as possible.

Family Affliction	Associated Screening Test
Cancers	
Breast Cancer	Mammograms each year beginning at age 30. Self-examination for lumps. CEA and CA 15-3 blood tests
Cervical and Vaginal Cancers	Annual Pap smear and pelvic exam commencing at age 20
Colon Cancer	Test annually for blood in the stool, starting at age 30. CEA blood test for carcinoembryonic antigen. Periodic colonoscopy. Annual proctosigmoidoscopy beginning at age 45. Rigid proctoscopy
Leukemia	Complete blood count, chromosome analysis, bone marrow biopsy
Lung Cancer	Annual chest x-ray and sputum exam beginning at age 50. NSE blood test
Oral Cancer	Annual dental examination. Biopsy
Ovarian Cancer, Cysts and Tumors	Annual pelvic exam. Ultrasonography. CA 125 blood test
Pancreatic Cancer	CA 19-9 blood test
Prostate Cancer	Digital rectal exam annually after age 40. PSA blood test that picks up presence of protein secreted by cancerous glands

Family Affliction	Associated Screening Test
Cancers (*continued*)	
Stomach Cancer	Periodic endoscopic examination, particularly if Barrett's syndrome is present
Testicular Cancer	AFP blood test for alpha-fetoprotein. Regular self examination. Ultrasound
Cancer of the Uterus	Endometrial biopsy
Other Diseases	
Cystic Fibrosis	Regular tests of lung function, stool and perspiration salinity
Diabetes	Blood-sugar test. Urinalysis
Glaucoma	Glaucoma exam at age 40
Heart Attack, Heart Disease, Atherosclerosis, Stroke	Regular blood pressure, serum cholesterol and triglyceride tests. Electrocardiogram. Exercise-tolerance test
Mood Disorders	Psychiatric evaluation when symptoms – chronic depression, major mood swings – first present themselves
Osteoporosis	Bone-density assessment before menopause
Polycystic Kidney Disease, Kidney Tumors	Urinalysis, ultrasound, CAT scan
Schizophrenia	Psychiatric evaluation when symptoms – delusions, hallucinations, incoherence – first present themselves

30 | Learn All You Can About The Diseases That Run In Your Family

If there is a familial pattern of medical problems in your clan, you should protect yourself by following the maxim, "Keep your friends close and your enemies closer still." You should know your enemy diseases inside out.

At the library, read up on the afflictions that pose a threat to you. Because of ever-occurring advances in research and treatment, look for the most recently published, up-to-date volumes. Too, you should keep up with news of research developments and findings. Use press reports of advances wisely, though — as notification to seek the medical journal that is the probable source of the press coverage. The general press generally sensationalizes and oversimplifies medical-research findings and often reports them inaccurately; the professional journal can give you the detailed information you need, appropriately leavened with all the necessary caveats and qualifications.

By becoming a lay expert, you know what symptoms to look for, you learn what procedures can best treat the disease, and you become familiar with the medical terminology. You can then also converse knowledgeably with your doctor about the matter.

Your doctor is there to serve your medical needs. Be sure you use her as an information resource. Ask questions about what concerns you. Tap your physician for the latest developments concerning your diseases of interest. Discuss what *both* of you can do to monitor and preempt those diseases. Develop a screening program.

As important, your knowledge enables you to look over your doctor's shoulder. That not only ensures she is paying appropriate attention to your concerns but also protects your interests should your alertness catch something the doctor missed. For more information about reducing the risks the medical establishment itself can pose for your longevity, please see Chapter 6.

You may also benefit by joining or contributing to an association or self-help group that combats the disease most prevalent in your family history. Information, advice about screenings and support services are some of the benefits you can hope to get from contacting such an organization. Table 3-3 lists some of the leading organizations and self-help clearinghouses for common disorders.

Table 3-3 | Organized for Battle

The organizations listed below are concerned about and work to combat major diseases and/or their effects.

Alzheimer's Association, 919 North Michigan, 10th Floor, Chicago, IL 60611; 312-335-8700

American Association of Kidney Patients, 111 South Parker Street, Suite 405, Tampa, FL 33606; 813-251-0725

American Cancer Society, 1599 Clifton Road, N.E., Atlanta, GA 30329; 404-320-3333

American Diabetes Association, National Center, P.O. Box 25757, 1660 Duke Street, Alexandria, VA 22314; 703-549-1500

American Heart Association, 7272 Greenville Avenue, Dallas, TX 75231; 214-373-6300

(continued)

Table 3-3 | Organized for Battle (*continued*)

American Kidney Fund, 6110 Executive Boulevard, Suite 1010, Rockville, MD 20852; 301-881-3052

American Brain Tumor Association, 3725 North Talman Avenue, Chicago, IL 60618; 312-286-5571

Cancer Control Society, 2043 North Berendo Street, Los Angeles, CA 90027; 213-663-7801

Candlelighters Childhood Cancer Foundation, 1312 18th Street, N.W., #200, Washington, DC 20036; 202-659-5136

Cystic Fibrosis Foundation, 6931 Arlington Road, #200, Bethesda, MD 20814; 301-951-4422

Huntington's Disease Society of America, 140 West 22nd Street, 6th Floor, New York, NY 10011; 212-242-1968

Leukemia Society of America, 733 Third Avenue, New York, NY 10017; 212-573-8484

Mended Hearts, 7320 Greenville Avenue, Dallas, TX 75231; 214-706-1442

National Depressive and Manic Depressive Association, 730 North Franklin, Suite 501, Chicago, IL 60610; 312-642-0049

National Digestive Diseases Information Clearinghouse, Box NDDIC, 9000 Rockville Pike, Bethesda, MD 20892; 301-468-6344

National Hypertension Association, 324 East 30th Street, New York, NY 10016; 212-889-3557

National Kidney Foundation, 30 East 33rd Street, New York, NY 10016; 212-889-2210

National Osteoporosis Foundation, 2100 M Street, N.W., Suite 602, Washington, DC 20037; 202-223-2226

Self-Help Clearinghouses in the U.S.

California*	800-222-LINK (CA only)
	For verification call 310-825-1799
Connecticut	203-789-7645
Illinois*	708-328-0470
	For administrative call 708-328-0471
Iowa	800-383-4777 (IA only)
	515-576-5870
Kansas	800-445-0116 (KS only)
	316-689-3843
Massachusetts	413-545-2313
Michigan*	800-777-5556 (MI only)
	517-484-7373
Minnesota	612-224-1133
Missouri (Kansas City)	816-472-HELP
Missouri (St. Louis)	314-773-1399
Nebraska	402-476-9668
New Jersey	800-FOR-MASH (NJ only)
	201-625-9565
New York (Brooklyn)	718-875-1420
New York (Westchester)**	914-949-6301
North Carolina (Mecklenberg area)	704-331-9500
Ohio (Dayton area)	513-225-3004
Oregon (Portland area)	503-222-5555
Pennsylvania (Pittsburgh area)	412-261-5363
Pennsylvania (Scranton area)	717-961-1234
South Carolina (Midlands area)	803-791-9227

(continued)

Table 3-3 | **Organized for Battle** (*continued*)

Tennessee (Knoxville area)   615-584-6736

Tennessee (Memphis area)   901-323-0633

Texas*   512-454-3706

Greater Washington, DC   703-941-LINK

---

*maintains listings of additional local clearinghouses operating within
  that state

**call Westchester only for referral to local clearinghouses in upstate
  New York

For national U.S. listings and directories:

American Self-Help Clearinghouse   201-625-7101

                                                                  TDD 201-625-9053

                                                                  FAX 201-625-8848

National Self-Help Clearinghouse   212-642-2944

Source: American Self-Help Clearinghouse, July 1992.

4 | Safety

Are you in the habit of consulting a daily horoscope? Do you believe there's a calendar in the Great Somewhere that has the date of your death circled in red?

If you answered yes, you may think accidents are largely a matter of fate.

In fact, accidents are predetermined, but not by fate. It is *we* who carelessly go about setting up the optimal conditions to make accidents happen: We drink alcohol and drive; we leave toddlers unattended in the bathtub; we overreach atop 30-foot ladders to apply that last spot of paint to the house trim.

The good news is, *we* can also carefully go about making accidents not happen.

By so doing, we can take major strides toward the 100-year mark, because accidents are the fourth-leading cause of death in the United States. They claim some 96,000 lives each year and inflict another 9.1 million disabling injuries.

On average, eliminating all accidents would add only about a year to the hypothetical U.S. life expectancy, according to the National Center for Health Statistics (NCHS). But if the people who were killed in accidents had somehow been able to avoid their fatal encounters, they would have added an average 23 to 38 years to their lives. That's nothing to sneeze at.

Here's what you can do to start bankrolling those bonus years.

31 | Buy a Car You Wouldn't Mind Wrecking

Most people buy a car because it's sexy or sporty looking, or because it parks nicely into a tight budget. But if you're serious about blowing out 100 birthday candles someday, get right down to business: Choose a car you wouldn't mind smashing into a tree.

Motor-vehicle accidents account for more than half of all accidental deaths, claiming some 49,000 lives each year. If there's a chance you could be involved in a fatal wreck—and there is—you want to be in a crashworthy vehicle.

With apologies to environmentalists everywhere, that means the bigger, more massive your car, the better your chances of surviving a crack-up are. When U.S. automobiles lost width and shed 1,000 pounds in the late 1970s to early 1980s, they became more fuel efficient but they also became deadlier. According to the National Highway Traffic Safety Administration, automobile downsizing added 2,000 fatalities and 20,000 serious injuries to the annual highway death toll.

That makes a compelling argument against buying a temptingly inexpensive compact. Even if it breaks the budget, a larger, more expensive car may be a good investment in your future—literally.

According to the Highway Loss Data Institute (HLDI), smaller cars generate greater injury claims than larger cars. HLDI uses an index in which 100 is the average loss for all cars. Ratings below 100 indicate losses are lower than average; ratings above 100 represent greater-than-average losses. For example, HLDI data show that all two-door large cars generate a rating of 91 in injury losses, while midsize models get 109, and small cars hit 132. Large luxury cars score best, with a 61 rating, followed by large four-door models, with a 65 rating. Table 4-1 lists the best and worst injury-loss ratings among popular car models.

But there's more to the science of crashworthiness than just sheer mass. The safest cars are specifically designed to withstand a crash. Take the Mercedes S-class car, whose design is based on 10 years of systematic real-world accident investigation and is highly rated in our table. It uses plenty of heavy metal to safely cocoon passengers.

Its structural framing diverts impact forces around the passenger compartment and away from passengers; breakaway engine mounts and chassis are designed to shove the engine underneath the passenger compartment instead of through it in a crash; strong roof pillars protect against rollovers; and a heavy rear firewall stands between people and the exploding gas tank that could result from a rear-end collision.

Crumple zones – empty spaces under a car's hood, where impact energies can be safely absorbed before they get into the passenger compartment – are also important. That's why you're less safe in a van or minivan (with virtually no hood between impact obstacle and front passengers) than you are sitting behind the bowling-alley-length hood of a Cadillac Fleetwood. (And needless to say, if you own a motorcycle – which offers no crash protection at all – junk that suicide machine.)

To get annual HLDI accident-loss ratings on more than 100 car models, send a self-addressed, stamped envelope to: Insurance Institute for Highway Safety, P.O. Box 1420, Arlington, VA 22210.

Fay Alexander believes she's lived to 105 because, in her own words, "I led a clean life – that's the only kind of life to live." She also believes being conscious about safety when driving had added years to her life. But this former print-shop worker has a genetic advantage working in her favor, as well. While her father died at 75 and her mother at 85, Fay's sister Leisha is also over 100 and her grandmother died when she was "almost 100."

Table 4-1 | Best and Worst Car Models

Listed below are the car models with actual overall accident-injury losses rated substantially better than average and the car models with actual overall accident-injury losses rated substantially worse than average by the Highway Loss Data Institute. Ratings are for 1988-90 models. The rating scale ranges from 37 (safest) to 184.

Rank	Make, Model, Description, Size	Rating
Better than average		
1	Chevy Caprice 4D, Large	37
2	Volvo 740/760 Station Wagon, Midsize	44
3	Jaguar XJ6 Luxury, Large	47
	Lexus LS400 Luxury, Large	47
4	Mercedes SEL/SDL Luxury, Large	49
5	BMW 735i Luxury, Large	55
6	Plymouth Grand Voyager Station Wagon, Large	56
	Lincoln Continental Luxury, Midsize	56
7	Mercury Grand Marquis 4D, Large	57
8	Dodge Grand Caravan Station Wagon, Large	59
	Cadillac Fleetwood/Deville 4D Luxury, Large	59
	Lincoln Town Car Luxury, Large	59
9	Ford Crown Victoria 4D, Large	61
10	Dodge Caravan Passenger Van, Large	64
	Oldsmobile 98 4D, Large	64

(continued)

Table 4-1 | **Best and Worst Car Models** (*continued*)

Rank	Make, Model, Description, Size	Rating
Worse than average		
1	Hyundai Excel 2D, Small	184
2	Hyundai Excel 4D, Small	173
3	Nissan Sentra 2D, Small	164
4	Dodge Daytona 2D, Small	147
	Geo Storm 2D, Small	147
5	Chevy Cavalier 2D, Midsize	146
6	Ford Mustang Sports Car, Midsize	145
7	Ford Escort 2D, Small	142
8	Eagle Summit 4D, Small	139
9	Toyota Tercel 2D, Small	138
10	Mitsubishi Eclipse 2D, Small	137

Source: Highway Loss Data Institute

32 | Buy a Car With Airbags

Because of recent advances in automobile-safety technology, if you're in the market for a car, buy one that's just rolled off the

William B. Ellis, 100, of Cincinnati, Ohio, is practically a textbook case of "doing everything right." Throughout his life, he ate little red meat, never used salt, ate mostly whole-wheat bread and "plenty of fruits and vegetables." When he drives, he says he always wears his seat belt – and he's never had an accident. He believes in "early to bed, early to rise": He turns out the lights 9 p.m. and gets up the next day by 6:30 a.m..

Of course, no one is perfect. Bill was a smoker, but he managed to quit at age 80. What triggered this late-life turnabout? "I saw my brothers die in their 50s and 60s from smoking," he laments.

Unsatisfied with the pills for circulation that a doctor prescribed years ago, he simply threw them away and substituted vitamin E supplements instead. Combined with support and elevation for his legs, the pills work "just as well, if not better than, medicine," according to Bill.

His mental attitude may have a lot do with his longevity. "I learned a long time ago to walk away from trouble and to keep my opinions to myself," he says.

assembly line instead of a used one. Some of the latest models are significantly safer than used cars – even used cars that are only a couple of years old. One reason for this is that newer cars are more likely to have airbags.

Nearly 25,000 traffic deaths and 300,000 serious injuries per year are caused by front-end crashes. Airbags help prevent this by inflating explosively into a protective pillow in front of the driver (and front passenger, if the car is so equipped) in a moderate- to high-speed frontal crash. The National Highway Traffic Safety Administration says that by the next decade, when all cars have airbags, 9,000 lives a year will be saved and 150,000 serious injuries will be prevented.

Airbags do not guarantee immortality, but when used in combination with seat belts, they significantly improve your chances of survival. According to a study by the Insurance Institute for Highway Safety, cars with airbags account for 28 percent fewer driver deaths than cars that have seat belts only.

By 1994 passive restraints for drivers and front passengers will be standard; most manufacturers are meeting this requirement with airbags. But until then, you can't assume the car you buy has them. Airbags tend to be standard on more-expensive models. Check Table 4-2 to see which cars have them. Also remember, some vehicles—light trucks, vans and multipurpose vehicles—are not yet required to have passive restraints.

33 | Buy a Car With an Antilock-Braking System

Another important safety feature your car should be equipped with is an antilock-braking system (ABS). An ABS gives a driver more control when she has to suddenly slam on the brakes on wet or slippery pavement. The ABS automatically pumps the brakes to prevent them from locking up and so helps the tires keep contact with the road.

The NHTSA hasn't yet determined how many lives could

be saved by ABS, but it recommends that automakers volun-
tarily install the $400 to $1,000 item on all cars. Only about
10 percent of new cars sold have ABS either as standard or
optional equipment. Generally, high-priced cars have ABS, but
GM says all its cars will have ABS standard by 1995. Refer to
Table 4-2 to see which carmakers offer the most cars with ABS
standard or optional now.

34 | Look for Stronger Sidewalls When You Buy a Car

Finally, because side collisions are the second-leading cause of
death and serious injury in motor-vehicle accidents—8,000
deaths and 24,000 serious injuries per year—federal regula-
tions have beefed up the standards for sidewall strength; by
1994 all new cars must meet them.

Some cars may already meet those standards because of
inherent design superiority. The bulky doors on large cars, for
example, afford slightly more crumple space and padding;
four-door models, which require a heavy steel center post,
offer greater protection than two-door models. When the sides
of all new cars are strengthened, an estimated 500 deaths and
2,600 serious injuries will be averted.

Other less-common safety features worth considering:
collapsible steering-wheel column, which is less likely to spear
you in a crash; built-in child safety seats; and independent
four-wheel-drive systems that sense wheel slippage and apply
differential power to each wheel, as appropriate, to pull you
out of a skid.

Table 4-2 | Airbags and ABS

The table below shows the percentage of manufacturers' 1991 sales volume with antilock-braking systems (ABS); driver airbags listed are on 1992 models. Optional driver airbags are denoted with "DO."

Acura
ABS: 65%
Airbags: Legend; NSX

Audi
ABS: 85%
Airbags: All models

BMW
ABS: 100%
Airbags: All models

Chrysler/Dodge/ Eagle/Plymouth
ABS: 4%
Airbags: Acclaim; Caravan; Daytona; Dynasty; Grand Caravan; Grand Voyager; Imperial; LeBaron; New Yorker; Shadow; Spirit; Stealth; Sundance; Voyager

Ford/Lincoln/Mercury
ABS: 17%
Airbags: Aerostar; Capri; Continental; Crown Victoria; Lincoln (all models); Grand Marquis; Mustang; Sable; Taurus; Tempo (DO); Topaz (DO); Town Car

GM/Buick/Cadillac/ Chevrolet/Geo/ Oldsmobile/ Pontiac/Saturn
ABS: 24%
Airbags: Cadillac (all models except Brougham); Chevrolet Beretta; Chevrolet Camaro; Chevy Caprice; Chevy Corsica; Chevy Corvette; Olds Custom Cruiser; Pontiac Bonneville; Pontiac Firebird; Geo Metro; Olds 88; Olds 98; Buick LaSabre; Buick Park Avenue; Buick Riviera; Buick Roadmaster; Geo Storm; Olds Toronado

Honda
ABS: 5%
Airbags: Accord; Civic

Infiniti
ABS: 100%
Airbags: M30; Q45

Isuzu
ABS: None
Airbags: All models

Jaguar
ABS: 100%
Airbags: XJ-S

Mazda
ABS: 10%
Airbags: MX-5 Miata;
RX-7 Convertible; 929

Mercedes-Benz
ABS: 100%
Airbags: All models

Mitsubishi
ABS: 13%
Airbags: 3000GT; Diamante

Nissan
ABS: 20%
Airbags: 300ZX; Maxima;
Sentra Coupe

Porsche
ABS: 100%
Airbags: All models

Saab
ABS: 100%
Airbags: All models

Subaru
ABS: 18%
Airbags: Legacy; SVX

Toyota
ABS: 9%
Airbags: Camry; Celica; Lexus;
Previa; Supra

Volkswagen
ABS: 6%
Airbags: Cabriolet

Volvo
ABS: 100%
Airbags: All models

Source: National Highway Traffic Safety Administration; Insurance Institute
for Highway Safety.

35 | Drive Like a Good Boy- Or Girl Scout

Of course, it goes without saying that safe driving begins with following the rules of the road and using common sense. Unfortunately, since too many others don't drive sensibly, you must drive defensively. That means practicing what you learned to do in Scouts: Be prepared.

Defensive driving revolves around the assumption that other drivers cannot be trusted to do what they're supposed to do. When that happens, a defensive driver has already anticipated the error and compensated accordingly. For example, a non-defensive driver sails through a green traffic light without care. A defensive driver doesn't stop either, but he keeps a wary eye on both sides of the crossroad for the remote possibility that someone will run the red light.

Defensive driving also involves recognizing and avoiding obvious road hazards—an aggressive driver intent on cutting you off and forcing you out of the way; a beat-up old jalopy with bald tires, crumpled fenders and plywood where the left rear window glass should be. Most drunk drivers can be found on the highway between 10 p.m. Saturday and 2 a.m. Sunday—a good time to be anywhere else.

Drivers at both ends of the age spectrum deserve special attention. Wild, young hot-rodders are dangerous; that's why the fatal-accident rate for drivers ages 15 to 24 is twice the norm. Give older drivers an extra safety margin, too, because their vision and hearing may be less than adequate and their reflexes slower. The fatal-accident rate for drivers age 75 and up is almost as bad as the young whippersnappers' rate.

Big rental trucks should be given a wide berth, as well, because it can be presumed the driver is inexperienced with such a large vehicle; the same might be said for the operators of mammoth recreational vehicles. Drivers pulling boats, housetrailers or cars-in-tow should be approached cautiously because they might not properly understand the length of their rigs or the extra requirements of navigating them. Monstrous buses, trucks, double tractor trailers and triple trailers need more elbowroom to maneuver, pick up speed and stop. And anytime you see a vehicle with something tied to the top of it or perched in a trailer, assume the darn thing is going to fly off and sail right at you like an ax in a 3-D horror movie.

36 | Don't Mix Driving and The Seven Dwarfs

You know the drill about drinking and driving, and even though half of all highway deaths are still caused by drunk drivers, we're not going to repeat the chorus about designated drivers and mocktails.

But another way drivers can make themselves Dopey — often without realizing it — is with prescription and over-the-counter medications. Whenever you're on any medication, be mindful of how the drug can slow your reflexes and induce drowsiness. If the drug impairs your abilities, don't drive. Tranquilizers — of course — can do this, but so can less obvious medications, such as muscle relaxants, antidepressants, antihistamines, blood pressure medicines and even powerful cold and flu remedies. Don't play Doc; consult your physician or pharmacist about the potential dangers.

Don't drive Sleepy either. There are no Mothers Against Drowsy Drivers, but an overtired driver can suffer the same handicaps as a drunk driver – blurred vision, poor judgment, slow reflexes, white-line fever (becoming hypnotized by the monotony of the night road) and the bizarre urge to curl up with a comfy-cozy steering wheel and sleep. The usual "antidotes" – strong coffee, caffeine tablets – only mask the symptoms of fatigue and may actually add to the probability of an accident. Worst times for driver fatigue: 3 p.m. to 2 a.m.

What about the other Dwarfs? People who are Grumpy, Sneezy with cold or flu, or (as mentioned) intoxicated from the Happy hour, are all at greater risk of having accidents, various studies show.

And don't be Bashful; according to *Sportsmanlike Driving*, a book published by the American Automobile Association in 1948, a person who is shy and retiring outside the car may become a monster once he gets behind the wheel of the great equalizer, to "give an artificial boost to his poor little self-esteem."

37 | Make Your Home In-*Fall*-ible

Believe it or not, falls are the number-two cause of accidental death. Most of these falls are not the kind you might expect – falling off the roof of your house while adjusting the antenna or bungee jumping with a loose bungee cord. Rather, these fatal falls come from seemingly innocuous household accidents: tripping over a rug, slipping in the shower, tumbling down the stairs.

For that reason – as with most accidents – potential victims can take precautions and eliminate the most common causes of falls. Getting rid of tripping hazards is especially important for older people because 70 percent of victims are age 65 and up. If the fall itself doesn't kill, a resulting disabling injury, such as a broken hip, could set in motion a long downward spiral in health.

Here's what you can do to avoid taking that first wrong step down the slippery slope:

•Secure throw rugs by taping them to the floor with double-sided stick tape (available at hardware stores) or by tacking them down.

•Repair worn stairs, frayed or torn stair runners, or crumbling outdoor concrete stairs. Install solid handrails along stairways, preferably on both sides. Install three-way switches that allow you to turn on lights from the top or bottom of staircases. Shovel off snow, then salt exterior stairways in cold weather. Be extra careful on steeply inclined basement stair-ways. If you're changing houses, eliminate stairs altogether by buying a single-level dwelling.

•In the bathroom, install sturdy handrails near tub, shower and toilet. Use stick-on appliques to create nonstick surfaces on the tub and shower floor. Make sure bathroom floor mats have rubber nonslip bottoms, or—better yet—install wall-to-wall carpeting.

•Around the house, wear slippers, sneakers or loafers that provide good traction and protect bare feet from sharp objects.

•Put modern technology to work. Get a cordless telephone and/or answering machine to eliminate the need for you to run to answer the phone. Use the clapper device (as seen on TV) that lets you turn lights on or off with a clap of your hands. Consider infrared sensors or motion detectors that can turn on lights automatically indoors or out at night when they sense your presence. Keep a lamp near your bed. Purchase a wireless battery-operated intercom so you needn't rush to answer your door.

• Remove clutter and excess furniture from around the house. Be sure electric cords don't stretch across walkways. And make sure those confounded pets don't get dangerously underfoot.

38 | Make Poisons Adult-Proof

Most safety advice concerning poisoning focuses things like on making sure toddlers don't chugalug sweet-tasting automobile antifreeze or make a snack of Drano crystals. The recommended precautions – safety locks on kitchen, garage and basement toxic-chemical cabinets, tamper-resistant caps on medicines and "Mr. Yuk" stickers on containers of poisonous materials – are well worth following, because children under age six suffer the greatest exposure to poisons, even though rates of death from poisoning are relatively low for this group. In 1987, for example, there were 732,000 poisoning exposures among children, resulting in 22 deaths and 108,000 nonfatal ill effects, according to the American Association of Poison Control Centers.

According to National Safety Council statistics, however, most poisoning fatality victims are not toddlers – they're adults! More than 60 percent of all people who die from poisoning by solids, liquids or gases are ages 25 to 44 (see Table 4-3). Those are the very same people who make sure the little tykes are not ingesting poisons and who are presumably the most poison-aware. By comparison, only 2 percent of poisoning fatalities are comprised of victims age 4 or younger.

How do 6,300 adults come to be poisoned each year? According to a study by the Centers for Disease Control, the leading culprits (in 27 percent of unintentional poisoning deaths) are illicit drugs—heroin, cocaine and other narcotics—which are clearly being abused. But another 34 percent of fatal poisonings result from prescription and over-the-counter drugs—antidepressants, antibiotics, nonnarcotic analgesics, cardiovascular drugs, acetaminophen and even aspirin. (These deaths result from an unknown combination of abuse, innocent accidental overdose, drug interactions, allergic reactions and drug-alcohol interactions; excluded are suicides and deaths related to drug dependence.)

Table 4-3 | Is Mr. Yuk Reaching All the "Kids"? (Annual Poisoning Fatalities By Age—1988)

When you think poison, you think young children. But actually, most victims of poisoning death are grown-ups.

Age-Group	Number of Poisoning Deaths
0 - 4	110 X
5 - 14	90 X
15 - 24	600 XXXXXX
25 - 44	3,800 XXXXXXXXXXXXXXXXXXXXXXXXXXXXXXXXXXXXXXXX
45 - 64	1,050 XXXXXXXXXXX
65 - 74	270 XXX
75+	380 XXXX

Source: National Safety Council.

Rose Ann Soloway, education coordinator for the National Capital Poison Center at Georgetown University, recommends adults take the following precautions:

• If you are using street drugs or abusing prescription or over-the-counter medications, you should seek professional help immediately, either from your physician or a hospital drug-treatment unit. If the drugs themselves don't kill you through overdose or adverse physical reaction, your addiction and continually drugged state can conspire against you to make some other accidental death much more likely. All of this is not to mention the devastating damage the drugs do to your body and longevity.

• Whenever you're on medications, don't use alcohol. Most drugs that affect the central nervous system have an exaggerated effect when alcohol is added. In general, it may take surprisingly little alcohol to create a dangerous interaction.

• Treat all drugs with proper respect. Read labels. Use them only for their intended purposes. Don't exceed prescribed dosages. Don't use someone else's prescription medicine. Don't store ingestible drugs in the medicine cabinet next to drugs not meant for ingestion. To avoid drug-to-drug interactions, whenever your doctor prescribes medicine, make her aware of any other prescription or over-the-counter drugs you are taking. Ask your pharmacist about possible drug interactions when you get your prescription filled. Don't assume any drug is safe; in large enough doses, even simple aspirin and acetaminophen can be lethal.

Two nondrug causes of poisoning merit words of caution. Every year there are news stories about fraternity hazings gone wrong because pledges consumed a large amount of alcohol in an extremely short period of time. Some 6 percent of unintentional poisoning fatalities are due directly to alcohol ingestion. Don't ever rise to the challenge of a stupid alcohol-consumption dare. Another 8 percent of deaths come from vehicular carbon-monoxide poisoning; never sit inside a closed garage with your car running, never warm up your car in a garage attached to your house and beware of carbon-monoxide leaks inside the passenger compartment of your car.

39 | Don't Mix Alcohol, Boats And Bathing Suits

Certain kinds of drownings get all the press coverage: toddlers in backyard pools, diving accidents, people who fall through thin ice and victims drawn to watery graves by flood-stage torrents. Those deaths are testament to commonsense wisdom: Don't leave young children unattended near water, never dive into waters of unknown depth, avoid swift river currents, don't venture onto frozen bodies of water unless you are certain the ice is thick enough to hold you, and take special precautions in inclement weather.

But there is another large class of drowning deaths that seemingly make no sense: Healthy, physically fit males and females in the company of friends who fall off boats, quietly drop beneath the water's surface on beautiful summer days, and never come back up.

Blame that demon rum—yet again. More than half of all boating deaths are alcohol related. Boaters who have been on the water exposed to sun, glare, wind, noise and vibration from the motor, and other motion develop fatigue after only four hours. Slowed reaction time while under the influence of boater's fatigue makes them as good as drunk without a drop of liquor.

Adding alcohol intensifies the effect, dulling the sense of balance. On the rolling deck of a boat, it suddenly becomes easy to tumble overboard.

Once in the water, alcohol incapacitates these people — whether they're already suffering from boater's fatigue or drinking alcohol while swimming at the beach. The alcohol in their blood makes them prone to overexposure to the cool waters much quicker than normal. A disorienting condition called *caloric labyrinthitis* distorts their sense of up and down when water enters their ear canals. A drunk can thus mistakenly believe he's swimming upward when in fact he's swimming down to Davy Jones' locker. And that is how many seemingly healthy boaters and swimmers disappear without a trace.

The solution: Never mix swimming with alcohol consumption, and keep alcohol off of boats.

40 | Don't Fight Fire Like Schwarzenegger

Each year more than a half-million home fires occur in the United States; they succeed in claiming some 5,000 lives. Most fires occur between 10 p.m. and 6 a.m., and the victims die of smoke inhalation and poisonous gases long before the flames get them. Part of the problem, says the National Safety Council, is that because of Hollywood mythmaking people just don't understand how deadly dangerous fire can be.

For example, because of thick black smoke, you cannot see well when inside a burning building the way a motion-picture camera appears to. (If moviemakers filmed fires realistically, you wouldn't be able to see what was going on.) On the big screen, fire moves slowly so that the hero has

plenty of time to save everyone; in real life, fire spreads very
rapidly. And movie stars can brave blasts of flame and still
make it out of a building with only sweat and grime to show
for their trouble – thanks to stunt doubles in fireproof suits; in
reality the intense radiant heat of a fire can fuse your clothes
to your body and make the air so hot it can sear your lungs.

Don't be fooled into thinking you can endure a fire the
way Arnold Schwarzenegger can. The best way for us mere
mortals to fight fire is to stop it before it starts:

• It seems almost ridiculously obvious, but be careful with
your cancer sticks. Almost 30 percent of all home fire deaths
are caused by just that. Frequently, a smoker in the living
room drops a cigarette onto the upholstery, where it smolders
undetected for hours. Later that evening, it suddenly bursts
into flames. If you need to smoke, stay off the couch, armchair
and bed.

• There are plenty of tips concerning safety precautions
when using portable heaters, which are the number-one cause
of fires and the second leading cause of fire fatalities. But we
like this bit of advice best: Don't use portable heaters. If the
heat in a particular room is inadequate, hunt down and block
draft sources, wear toasty socks and sweaters, or extend your
home's regular heating system into the room. When calculating
the cost of the new installation, be sure to add the price of
your and your family's lives to the cost of that seemingly less-
expensive portable heating alternative; you'll probably find the
permanent and safe installation is a lot less expensive.

• Install smoke detectors on each floor of your home – they
save lives – and map out primary and backup fire-escape routes
from each room. Smoke-detector batteries should be checked
twice a year; make it a habit to do it when you change your
clock backward or forward. You may feel corny, but periodically hold a fire drill so everyone understands what to do and
where to go in case of a fire.

41 | Treat Firearms Responsibly

Ownership of firearms is a constitutional right. But with that right comes the responsibility to ensure that guns are handled safely at all times and that they never be allowed to accidentally discharge, injure or kill. Accidental deaths from firearms number 1,400 a year. Add this to the number of murders committed with firearms—more than 11,000 a year—and you have a significant deterrent to long life sitting in your home.

To ensure gun safety at home, where 54 percent of gun accidents happen, the National Safety Council recommends the following:

• All firearms should be kept unloaded, secured with a trigger lock and locked away out of sight of children. Ammunition should also be locked away—in a place separate from the firearms. Some 250 accidental firearm deaths per year involve children age 14 or younger.

• Whenever guns are kept in the home, all members of the family should be educated in firearm safety. Even a spouse who may be politically and morally opposed to guns should learn about gun safety; what a person doesn't know about guns can hurt them and others. Children, especially, should be schooled in gun safety. This training starts with the example you set. Firearms should always be treated with strict care and respect; children usually learn by watching. Children should also be taught that firearms are not toys and that the make-believe shootouts they see in movies and on TV would be deadly real in their own homes. Finally, when children are old enough, they should be enrolled in a sportsmen's training course available at local gun clubs and firing ranges.

L.N. of LaFontaine, Indiana, is one determined lady. She's made it to 100, she says, by "deciding not to die." That strength of mind is what kept her going during 50 years of schoolteaching at all levels – an accomplishment in which she still takes justifiable pride. Because L.N. looked upon teaching as a personal calling, it gave her the sense of happiness and well-being so important to long life. After all, she says, "we all want to be happy."

L.N.'s determination may help to keep her well. She simply refuses to think about the kinds of accidents that often plague the elderly. "I'm too old to worry about things going wrong," she says.

5 | Environment

When Sue and Jim McCarthy moved into their new home in Jackson, New Jersey, in 1973, they felt they'd successfully secured their health and safety by getting out of polluted New York City. Two years later, though, the couple began experiencing chronic headaches, dizzy spells and dysentery. Their son Trevor developed skin rashes.

Then nine-month-old daughter Tara developed a rare form of kidney cancer and died in 1975. Two years later, one of Jim's kidneys atrophied and had to be removed. Two more years later, the family collie died. Other families in the area suffered the same kinds of serious kidney problems.

The health problems and Tara's death, it turns out, were more than just coincidence or a streak of bad luck; they flowed from the water faucet. The McCarthys' well water had been contaminated by a toxic-waste dump located about a mile from their home. Some 100,000 gallons of household, septic and chemical wastes were being indiscriminately dumped into the landfill each day. From there, poisons trickled down into the aquifer that the McCarthys' well had tapped, traveled up to the house and poured out the faucet. Subsequent testing found that, for years, each sparkling glass of water the McCarthys drank was invisibly tainted with 38 toxic chemicals—some carcinogenic (cancer-causing).

The McCarthys' experience is just one tragic example of how environmental hazards can sneak into someone's life and reduce that person's chances of ever getting close to old age. But it is not by any means an isolated incident. Environmental hazards—both manmade and natural—are a modern-day fact of life that can be extremely hazardous to your health. Because these threats can often be fatal, tomorrow's centenarians need to assess environmental dangers and take precautionary steps today.

Here are the potentially deadly dangers you should be on guard against:

42 | Unseal Your House to Flush Out Indoor Air Pollutants

When most people think air pollution, they point to factory smokestacks, tailpipes of city buses or solid-waste incinerators. Subconsciously, we associate air pollution with the great out-doors. However, some of the worst levels of air pollution can be found indoors, right in our own homes.

Like the smoky caves and thatched huts of our ancestors, our homes bottle up and concentrate any airborne pollutants generated by the inhabitants. Unfortunately, the modern American home does a much more efficient job of trapping pollutants than the cold and drafty habitats of the past.

The typical home designed to keep heat in and cold out still has enough cracks and gaps to permit its entire volume of air to be exchanged with the fresh outdoor air about once every hour. In the energy conscious '80s, however, we caulked, weatherstripped and plugged up the leaks. Breezy windows and doors were replaced by much more tightly sealed models. So-called supertight houses, built new, all but put a plastic bag over the homeowner's head. They can reduce air exchange to as little as one-tenth of the volume of the house per hour, according to *Consumer Reports* researchers.

That mightn't be so bad except for the fact that our homes are filled with scores of tiny pollution generators: aerosol sprays, cigarettes, toxic chemical fumes, even air conditioners and humidifiers.

Most indoor pollutants can take a long time before revealing their impact on the body, but they are deadly nonetheless. Even when indoor pollutants don't kill outright, they can have a detrimental and sometimes chronic impact on health, an unnecessary obstacle in your pathway to long life.

What can you do to eliminate this threat? Generally, it's a good idea not to seal up your house like a Thermos bottle. Your house is probably too tight if condensation forms on the windows during the winter, if there are mold and mildew on walls and ceilings, if odors linger and if your family suffers frequent respiratory problems. If you went overboard with the caulking gun, undo some of your handiwork and allow a few drafts here and there. Keeping the windows open as much as possible in spring, summer and fall flushes out pollutants and reduces your overall exposure to indoor pollution to only the coldest months of the year. And filling your house with plants provides natural air scrubbers that also soak up carbon dioxide and provide fresh oxygen.

43 | Banish Cigarette Smoke From Your Home

Ideally, cigarette smoke should be banished from your home entirely. Sidestream cigarette smoke may not seem to have an effect during years of exposure, but it increases a nonsmoker's risk of lung cancer by 30 percent. Use the threat your bad habit poses to nonsmoking family members as an incentive to quit smoking yourself. If that's not possible, protect the health of your family by never smoking inside the house. If you must still smoke inside, confine your smoking to only one ventilated room. If that's too much to ask and you absolutely cannot alter your habits, some room air cleaners can filter smoke from the air, as can electrostatic-precipitator air cleaners, which give airborne particles an electric charge and then attracts them to a collection plate.

44 | Treat Chemical Fumes With Caution

Chemical fumes should be treated with caution, too; they are more dangerous than you may think. For example, the U.S. Consumer Product Safety Commission estimates that for every 1,000 25-to-70-year-olds who spend only three hours per year using paint stripper in a poorly ventilated room, three will develop cancer from the exposure. That's because of a key carcinogenic ingredient, methylene chloride, which is also found in spray paint, hairsprays and insecticides.

Laura Edwards, of Camden, Arkansas, takes absolutely no personal credit for her long life. "I eat what I want. I do whatever I want. Don't smoke. Don't drink whiskey. I eat sweets – but not a lot," the 100-year-old explains.

Growing up in the fresh air of the country and, later, in a small town may have helped a mite, Laura concedes. She also admits she might have to thank her credo: "Don't get angry. I avoid anger by remembering that everything will turn out well," she says. Then there's her family, a definite life-extender. "They've always been nice and good to me. I have a good family."

But while all of these factors may have contributed to her long life, Laura is still not satisfied that she's given credit where credit is due. Then she knows: "God," she smiles contentedly. "God let me live this long."

Any products that produce chemical fumes – aerosol sprays, solvents, cleaners – should be used outdoors. When this is not possible, throw open the doors and windows to properly ventilate the house, using window fans blowing outward, if necessary. Try to use such products indoors only when outside temperatures are moderate, so the benefits of pollution control don't have to compete with the disadvantage of heat loss.

Air-conditioning systems and room humidifiers can be breeding grounds for pollutants, too – live pollutants, like fungi, bacteria and germs. Potentially fatal Legionnaires' disease can originate in air-conditioning equipment. Regularly clean and disinfect these devices and replace filters.

45 | Vent Household Combustion Appliances to the Outside

Each year, some 1,700 people die from asphyxiation due to carbon-monoxide poisoning in their homes, thanks to improperly vented heating and combustion devices. Dangerous levels of carbon monoxide, nitrogen dioxide, sulfur dioxide and particulates are produced by heating and cooking devices – gas stoves, kerosene space heaters, furnaces, fireplaces, wood stoves and gas hot-water heaters. If you have a garage attached to your home, pollutants from the car's engine can seep in, too.

A gas stove in a poorly ventilated kitchen can produce as much pollution as you would experience on a smog-alert day in Los Angeles. Carbon monoxide kills when enough molecules of it bind tightly to red blood cells and prevent them from carrying life-giving oxygen. That gaseous compound can also change heart rhythm. Nitrogen dioxide causes respiratory problems. Sulfur dioxide can set off asthma attacks.

Whenever you use a combustion device indoors, make sure its harmful gases are vented to the outdoors. The most likely violator of this rule is the kerosene space heater. Because of the fire hazard that is also associated with this appliance, in Chapter 4 we recommended you not use one at all. It makes absolutely no antipollution sense, either, to use an unvented combustion heater indoors. If you must use such a heater, however, stick the thing in your fireplace and vent it up the chimney. Make sure the heater is properly maintained and the wick properly adjusted. Crack open a window to allow a fresh-air flow.

Other combustion devices can deceive. Check your furnace to make sure the chimney is not blocked or otherwise constricted. An improperly drafted chimney can spew deadly gases into your house.

If you vent smoke or fumes out of a tightly sealed house with a fan, make sure you provide replacement-air inlets. Otherwise the furnace chimney could act as an inlet, and the resultant downdraft could pump carbon-monoxide gases from the furnace into the house.

In the kitchen, provide outside venting for the stove. Double-check your range-hood fan to make sure it vents outdoors. Some fans merely recirculate air through a filter and back into the kitchen; this does not filter out poisonous gases.

46 | If You Have a Garage Attached to Your House, Never Keep Your Car in It While the Engine Is Running

Even if your garage is detached, you should refrain from ever running the car in a completely closed garage. If you want to warm up the vehicle on cold mornings, consider an electric engine warmer or move the automobile out of the garage while the engine is warming.

When you drive your car into the garage, park it front first, so the tailpipe is closest to and sends exhaust outside through the open door, rather than pumping it into the confined spaces. After the car exits or enters the garage, leave the garage door open for several minutes so exhaust fumes can dissipate.

47 | Eliminate Radioactive Radon Gases From Your Home

In cigarette-free homes, some 5,000 to 20,000 lung-cancer deaths are caused each year by long-term exposure to radon gas, according to the U.S. Environmental Protection Agency. This naturally occurring radioactive gas seeps into homes from the ground below. The gas decays into elements called radon daughters, which attach to dust particles, are inhaled and lodge in the lining of the lungs. Over time, this exposure can cause cancer.

Have your house tested for the presence of radon gas – with "air-grab" samples, radiation-sensitive film detectors or continuously monitoring electronic detectors. As many as eight million U.S. homes may have a radon problem, says the EPA. Experts say all soil emits radon gas, not just soil in areas rich in subterranean uranium deposits, like the Reading Prong, which runs from eastern Pennsylvania through northern New Jersey and into southern New York. Contamination varies from house to house, depending on how underground rock and soil formations channel the gas. Inside a typical house, radon concentrations tend to be highest in the basement and progressively diminish on the first, second and upper floors.

If your house does have radon, you should seal cracks and openings in basement floors and walls where the gas may be entering, ventilate the basement or crawl space beneath your home, and/or ventilate the space beneath your basement floor. Heat-recovery ventilators can expel radon-laced air from your basement while retaining much of the indoor heat.

Another important preventive measure is to make sure devices that pump air out of your home have inlets that bring replacement air in from outside. For example, when your clothes dryer vents air to the outside, it creates a tiny vacuum inside your home by reducing indoor air pressure. When that happens, outside air – including radon-laced air in the ground beneath your home – gets sucked in through the cracks. Air inlets provide a ready flow of replacement air that helps maintain your indoor air pressure.

48 | Test Your Tap Water For Toxins

A wide variety of contaminants can get into your household water supply—toxic chemicals, many kinds of bacteria, lead. One study by Cornell University found that 63 percent of rural household water supplies are unsafe. The Environmental Protection Agency has found that 20 percent of public groundwater supply systems are contaminated with manmade pollutants; a third of the water systems serving larger communities are contaminated with chemicals.

The life-threatening danger from such contamination is real: cancers, birth defects, miscarriages, heart abnormalities, hepatitis, typhoid, convulsions, brain swelling, acute kidney disease, hypertension, hyperactivity, neurological abnormalities and reduced mental functioning.

The sources of contaminated water are abundant, too: landfills, toxic-waste dumps, manufacturers, underground gasoline tanks, septic tanks and even the lead pipes in your home. What should you do about the problem?

Have your water tested for contaminants at the tap. This is especially important if you get your water from your own well, because municipal water supplies are subject to regular monitoring and standards; your well is generally your responsibility.

Your local health department may test your well water for free or for a small fee. For about $100, you can have your water tested through a mail-order testing service, such as one listed in Table 5-1.

If your water is contaminated, you should switch to bottled water and contact your state or county health department to help hunt down the source. If the source is lead in your own home, you may have to replace the pipes.

Another solution is to install a water-filtration system for your potable-water needs. Activated-carbon filters are good for removing organic contaminants. They must be changed regularly, however, because eventually the filters become loaded with contaminants and begin dumping them into your glass. These filters are not useful against metal contamination.

A reverse-osmosis filter in combination with a carbon filter can remove just about all contaminants from water.

Table 5-1 | Testing the Waters

The mail-order companies listed below will test your tap water. Fees vary from $24.95 to $178, depending on how comprehensively you want your water tested.

National Testing Laboratories	800-458-3330
Suburban Water Testing Laboratories	800-433-6595

---

49 | Get in the Sunscreen Habit

A perpetually suntanned body is a sure sign of health, we have come to believe. But quite to the contrary, medical experts now warn, a suntan is an insult to the skin. For some 100,000 Americans per year, this insult leads to basal-cell carcinoma, a nonlethal skin cancer.

Another 100,000 people get squamous-cell cancer, a more aggressive skin neoplasm, but as successfully treated as basal-cell carcinoma—if detected early. The most serious form of skin cancer, malignant melanoma, strikes some 27,000 people each year. This aggressive, fast-spreading cancer kills about 25 percent of its victims and is dramatically on the rise, according to the American Cancer Society. Cause: depletion of atmospheric ozone (which screens us from harmful ultraviolet radiation) over northern New England, Canada, northern Europe and Russia.

Luckily, you don't have to cover yourself head to toe with clothing or shun daylight like Dracula to protect yourself. You merely have to take a few precautions.

Your risk of getting skin cancer is directly related to the amount of time you spend in the sun, so your best precaution is to limit your time in the sun—especially if you have a family history of skin cancer or are fair-skinned, fair-haired and blue-eyed. That means you should avoid intentionally sitting under the sun for the express purpose of getting a tan. Nor should you train a sunlamp on yourself or use a tanning parlor.

Skin cancer is set off by the sun's ultraviolet rays. Since these rays are strongest between 10 a.m. and 3 p.m., limit your exposure to the sun during those hours. If you must be out-doors at that time, use a sunscreen with a sun-protection factor (SPF) of 15, wear a wide-brimmed hat and consider long sleeves and pants for unsunscreened arms and legs. Apply sunscreen 30 minutes before going into sunlight, and reapply every 90 minutes or sooner if water, sweat, towels or clothing might have removed some of it.

The skin of children is particularly susceptible to sun-burn, exposing them to a greater risk of the worst type of skin cancer. According to studies at New York Hospital-Cornell Medical Center, young children exposed to only three bad sunburns have a three times greater chance of developing malignant melanoma in later years. For that reason, you should apply sunscreen liberally to the kiddies. Wherever possible around your house, set up shady play areas. At the beach use an umbrella or portable canopy.

You should also regularly examine your body markings and moles. A change in color, size, thickness or outline could be skin cancer announcing itself. Crusting and reopening sores that last for more than four weeks or are persistently itchy, bleeding or crusting are other warning signs. When any of these show up, immediately bring them to the attention of your physician. As with all cancers, early detection and treatment of skin cancer is the key to survival.

50 | Beware Your Likeliest Murderer: An Acquaintance

Every 20 seconds, a violent crime is committed in the United States – aggravated assault, robbery, rape, murder. Violent crime is a manmade environmental hazard. But while broad political and socioeconomic action is necessary to reduce and better control this hazard, you can take personal steps to control your exposure to this life-threatening danger.

When we think of being murdered, most of us conjure up ghoulish images of Ted Bundy grabbing us unawares or of a stranger picking us out at random. In fact, most murders are far from senseless acts of fate. The Federal Bureau of Investigation compiles information about the circumstances surrounding murder in the United States, and an analysis of the how and why of real murders can provide the valuable information you need to help reduce your chances of becoming a victim.

Data show that most victims know their murderers; in killings where a relationship can be determined, only about 18 percent of murderers are total strangers. The rest of the killers are people the victims knew. But who?

Statistics suggest you should keep your most wary eye on acquaintances – people you've met but don't know well – rather than friends, neighbors or family. Where the relationship between murderer and victim can be determined, acquaintances are responsible for 45 percent of all murders, as opposed to just 11 percent for spouses, 6 percent for boyfriends or girlfriends, 6 percent for friends and 2 percent for neighbors.

In murders related to romantic triangles, acquaintances commit 58 percent of the killings, suggesting that the interloper is the one to watch out for and that the movie *Fatal Attraction* is must viewing for every couple. Men with cheatin' hearts should especially beware: Wives or girlfriends are 3½ times more likely to act homicidal than husbands or boyfriends, committing 16.6 percent of such murders *vs.* only 4.8 percent for men. The weapon of choice is a gun (68 percent of the time), with cutting instruments second (20 percent).

Where the murder's cause is known, 44 percent of deaths result from arguments. To avoid such a fatal situation, learn to walk away from disputes whenever possible by refusing to let yourself get "hooked" into an argument. If a debate becomes heated, agree to disagree; talk about it later, after both sides have cooled down. Avoid provoking arguments, and if, despite your best efforts, an argument has developed, don't escalate it. Take any threats of violence as serious advice to back off. If you find you have a penchant for heated discussions or that you just seem to attract argumentative types, explore the psychological roots of this anger/hostility predisposition with a professional counselor or by reading books on the subject. The same advice can help you avoid episodes of aggravated assault.

Another 28 percent of murders take place as other felonies are being committed – primarily robbery and narcotics-related crime – so knowing how to avoid those types of crime could also save your neck.

It should go without saying that you should stay away from the use or sale of narcotics. Don't associate with anyone who uses or sells drugs.

The kind of robbery you're most likely to encounter is a street mugging (54 percent of all robberies are of this kind). Don't make yourself an attractive target by counting money in public or flaunting expensive jewelry or accessories. Women should keep their pocketbooks hugged close to their bodies. Don't withdraw cash from automated-teller machines late at night, and avoid poorly lit, desolate areas with landscape features that could seclude a violent criminal lying in wait. Police also advise that, whenever you're out and about, you walk with a head-high, confident attitude and be obviously aware of your surroundings; a head-down pedestrian who's lost in his own thoughts and doesn't have the faintest idea who's nearby is easy pickings for a robbery. For the same reasons, avoid being obviously intoxicated in public, when you're less alert, less sensitive to potential dangers and physically incapacitated.

It's wise to recognize the relative robbery risks of the different environments you travel in. You're at greatest risk of street robbery in the largest cities; 62 percent of urban robberies are street muggings. In contrast, in cities with populations under 10,000, only 26 percent of the robberies are street crimes; small-town crooks have a greater preference for robbing commercial establishments than their big-city cohorts. Robbery and other violent crimes are also higher in areas with high numbers of transients, which is why resort areas like

Las Vegas, Orlando and Atlantic City have high crime rates; the flood of tourists provides plenty of monied crime targets, and opportunistic criminal visitors easily blend in with the population ebbs and flows.

College students are especially vulnerable to crime because of the immortality mind set of youth and the misperception that crime doesn't take place on campus. Stick to well-lit pathways and know where emergency phones are located. Use escort and van services for night travel. Curb alcohol use, which, according to a study by Towson State University, is associated with 80 percent of campus rape, assault and vandalism. Be aware of campus crime rates. And, of course, lock dorm-room doors.

Robbery in the home is less likely, comprising only 10 percent of all robberies. Criminals prefer burglarizing a home when there's no one there, but it's possible you'll wind up staring down an assailant if you happen upon a robbery in progress. The best deterrents are good outdoor lighting, appropriate locks on doors and windows, and neighbors who keep watch over each other's property well enough to report suspicious characters. Block associations are a good way to bind community members to each other in this protective endeavor. In larger communities, police may offer residents an opportunity to participate in formal Crime Watch programs. Participants in such programs are specially trained to spot and report trouble in their neighborhoods.

What about the major violent-crime fear of women—the rape-murder? While the fear is understandable, the likelihood is not great. Rape rates may be skyrocketing, but only three-tenths of 1 percent of all murders are associated with sex offenses. Nevertheless, by following the advice given above for stopping other forms of violent crime, women can reduce their chances of being raped.

51 | Don't Live in Environmentally Hazardous Locales

Where you live plays an increasingly important part in how long you live. Air and water pollution, toxic-waste dumps, nuclear power plants, smog—potential life and health hazards all—can be found in every section of the United States. But you can dodge these dangers by carefully choosing the place you call home.

Before you settle on a home or area, find out who your "neighbors" are. Toxic-waste dumps—most concentrated in the Northeast—are of prime concern. Check with your state department of environmental resources for information about known dump sites in your county and region.

But be aware that some properties, while not officially designated as toxic-waste dumps, can also be polluted with toxins and should be avoided: military bases, weapons-manufacturing facilities, chemical companies, gas stations (because of leaking underground storage tanks), municipal landfills (even if they don't accept hazardous wastes), computer-component manufacturing plants, mining operations, oil refineries, any factory that uses chemicals in its production, and even farms (because of the constant use of pesticides and fertilizers).

Another potentially deadly neighbor is a nuclear power plant. Most U.S. atomic plants are located east of the Mississippi, particularly in Illinois, Pennsylvania, New Jersey and South Carolina. Are they life threatening? Regulators downplay the danger. Two people died in the explosion at the Chernobyl nuclear reactor in 1986, and 29 more from radiation sickness.

Wind currents spread radioactivity throughout Europe (exposing some 550 million people) and large parts of the former Soviet Union. Some 135,000 people were evacuated from contaminated areas surrounding the plant.

Experts predicted that the accident would create only about 7,000 new cases of cancer. But it will be years before scientists know the true effects of the disaster; the International Nuclear Energy Agency said it would monitor the 135,000 evacuees for the next 50 years. In 1991 medical experts reported a doubling of cancer rates, particularly of the lip and thyroid, in the areas surrounding the plant. Other reports noted: an increase in chronic illness in Chernobyl-area humans; high levels of radiation in area wildlife and genetic damage in rodents; and pine-tree needles growing 10 times their normal size.

Each year, U.S. nuclear plants experience about 3,000 "potentially significant safety accidents," according to the Nuclear Regulatory Commission. Because of the number of nuclear plants in the United States, the far-reaching potential for dispersal of radiation by wind currents and the unpredictability of a serious accident, no location is truly safe from a nuclear accident and it is impractical to try to escape. However, it is certainly advisable not to live in the immediate vicinity or downwind of such a facility, where contamination concentrations would likely be highest. A study conducted by a Columbia University epidemiologist shows that cancer rates in the area immediately surrounding the Three Mile Island nuclear reactor did not rise appreciably in the six years following its brief accident in 1979. But for people who were living directly in the path of the radioactive plume the plant spewed forth, there was an increased incidence of lung cancer and non-Hodgkin's lymphoma.

52 | If You're Considering A Relocation, Choose a City Or Town That Will Be Conducive To a Healthy Lifestyle

Some locations make it easier for you to lead a healthy lifestyle than others. If you are a person whose body responds strongly to stress, a high-pressured, fast-paced environment may not be for you. On the other hand, if you thrive on opportunities to explore a wide variety of exercise opportunities, you might want a big city with a wide variety of recreational opportunities. Table 5-2 lists 20 of the healthiest cities in America, based on author John Tepper Marlin's analysis of air and water quality, crime rate, life expectancy, health services, recreational opportunities and so forth.

53 | Eliminate Lead From Water, Walls and Dishware

A growing number of studies show that millions of Americans suffer from excessive levels of lead in their bloodstreams. Children are at greatest risk—from lead-caused kidney and neurological problems and intellectual impairment. But lead poisoning can create miscarriages, birth defects and premature birth, and middle-aged men can get hypertension from elevated lead levels in their blood.

Where does household lead come from? From some of the most unlikely places. Some 30 million homes still have old lead paint on the walls; when young, upwardly mobile home-owners remodel or renovate, the lead dust literally flies, to be inhaled or picked up from dusty surfaces.

Table 5-2 | The 20 Healthiest Cities in the U.S.

Are you fed up with pollution, crime and other factors in big-city life? Here are 20 cities where the quality of life may help you live longer.

---

1. Honolulu	11. Colorado Springs
2. Anchorage	12. Atlanta
3. Denver-Aurora-Boulder	13. Richmond
4. Charlotte	14. Minneapolis-St. Paul
5. Bridgeport-Stamford	15. Dallas-Ft. Worth
6. Washington, D.C.	16. Austin
7. Salt Lake City	17. Raleigh-Durham
8. Seattle	18. Boise
9. Miami-Hialeah	19. Des Moines
10. Sacramento	20. Houston

Source: The Livable Cities Almanac by John Tepper Marlin (New York: HarperCollins, 1992).

Homes near major highways can have high lead content thanks to years of leaded-gasoline exhaust fumes wafting over and depositing the metal on soil and household surfaces. When you store wine in a lead-crystal decanter or acidic foods in some imported ceramics, lead leaches out of the crystal or ceramic and into the wine or food. And some 40 million American homes have tap water containing dangerous amounts of lead, which leaches into the water from lead pipes and lead-solder pipe joints.

What should you do about it? Have your doctor administer the "Blood Lead Test" to family members, especially if children exhibit some of the symptoms of lead poisoning: mood swings, excessive crying, abdominal pains, slowed growth and irritability. (Of course, lead-free kids can show these same symptoms, too.) Lead-poisoned adults may suffer insomnia, crankiness, muscle pains, anemia, headaches and weight loss.

If high lead levels show up in the blood test, you must find the source. Contact the American Council of Independent Labs (129 K Street, N.W., Suite 400, Washington, DC 20006) to locate labs that test for lead. If the problem is lead paint, have a professional remove it with a chemical paint stripper. Don't sand it off, because the dust will only add to your exposure. Contaminated soil can be covered with concrete.

If your plumbing is the culprit, the expensive remedy is to replace the lead pipes. Less expensive is a lead filter to purify drinking water. Inexpensive cure: Flush the lead out of the water each day by running the faucet for three to five minutes each morning. Use only cold tap water for drinking and cooking, because lead is more likely to leach into hot in-the-pipes water.

To avoid lead poisoning from food vessels, never store wine in a lead-crystal decanter and don't use any imported ceramicware containing lead. Those contents tend to draw lead out of the crystal and ceramic.

54 | Unless It's Crumbling, Leave Asbestos Alone

For years now, homeowners have worried about the presence of asbestos in their homes. Workers who have been subject to long-term asbestos exposure do run an increased risk of cancer, but recent studies have concluded that low-level, short-term exposure to asbestos does not significantly increase a person's chances of getting lung cancer.

If you suspect there is an asbestos danger in your home, have the air tested for it. Your local health department should be able to provide you with names of state- and EPA-certified environmental services/contractors who can conduct such tests. In general, however, unless the asbestos is crumbling— *friable* in scientific jargon—the best remedy is to let it alone. When removal crews tear out asbestos, they can throw huge amounts of asbestos dust in the air. This can settle around the house and in air ducts, creating a bigger hazard than you had before.

55 | Eliminate Microbial Contamination From Food

The foods we eat can carry a number of microbial contaminants, including *salmonella*, *campylobacter* and other bacteria. A former assistant secretary of agriculture estimates that

85 percent of all poultry is contaminated with either salmonella or campylobacter, both of which can cause symptoms of food poisoning. In most cases, ingestion of these contaminants results in unpleasant, flulike symptoms: vomiting, abdominal pain, intestinal distress. But each year more than 2,000 people die from salmonella poisoning, and a rare strain of bacteria in undercooked beef has been known to produce a powerful poison that may attack the brain or result in kidney failure. Furthermore, a 1985 report by the National Academy of Sciences concluded that U.S. Department of Agriculture inspection procedures are not providing sufficient protection against unwholesome beef. Among the problems with meat are contamination by fecal matter, bacteria and the processing of sick and diseased cattle for market. The key to protecting yourself is to pay attention when you prepare, cook and handle food.

To combat microbials, assume all meat and poultry are contaminated and cook them thoroughly. Wash hands after handling meat so you don't spread contaminants to other foods that won't be cooked. Set the oven no lower than 325°F.; below that level bacteria can survive and multiply rapidly. Refrigerate leftovers promptly. Cook eggs thoroughly and don't use cracked eggs—because salmonella can enter the egg through the cracks.

56 | Protect Yourself Against Pesticide Contamination

It's a given that many of the pesticides used in this country have proven carcinogenic in tests with laboratory animals. But in most cases, experts disagree on the amount of exposure needed for human beings to suffer cancer. The best bet is to err on the side of caution by getting rid of as many pesticide residues as you can. To protect yourself from pesticides, wash all fruits and vegetables before using. A little vinegar or citric acid can help remove water-insoluble pesticides, but be aware that some pesticides always penetrate too deeply into the plant to be removed. You may want to remove the peels, outer leaves of lettuces and cabbages, and celery leaves to reduce pesticides further, but in many cases this also eliminates important nutritional value. A realistic alternative is to buy produce that's guaranteed organically grown without pesticides, or to grow your own. If neither of these is an option for you, at least buy from local growers, who can provide information about pesticide use before you buy.

57 | Choose and Treat Fish Carefully

Fish present even more problems. A 1992 examination by *Consumer Reports* researchers found that half the store-bought fish tested were contaminated with human or animal feces, and 40 percent were of only fair to poor quality, thanks to bacteria. An added danger with some fish and shellfish is toxic chemicals, since fish live in the waters we pollute. Fish can contain everything from the industrial pollutant PCB to the pesticide DDT, to lead, mercury and arsenic.

As with meats, assume the worst about fish and cook thoroughly. Shun raw seafood no matter how in vogue it may be. And use a wide variety of fish from different habitats, to reduce exposure to any one contaminant. Pregnant women should avoid fish while they're with child because of the pollutants.

58 | If You're in the Process Of Choosing an Occupation, Eliminate the Most Risky Ones Where Possible

Let's face it, if all you ever dreamed about was being a firefighter, it isn't practical to eliminate that from consideration simply because it's a very risky occupation. But if you're not wedded to a particular calling, it's worth considering that certain occupations lend themselves to long, healthy lives and some don't. While formal studies are scarce, researchers have noticed certain patterns.

For instance, most of us would consider the job of symphony conductor fairly stressful. Yet a 20-year study by the Metropolitan Life Insurance Company shows that the mortality rate for symphony conductors in different age-groups was, on average, 38 percent lower than for others in the same age-group. A separate study came up with similar findings for the very highest level of corporate executive. (Lower-level musicians and business executives had no such advantage.) And while "symphony conductor" or "CEO" may not necessarily be a realistic aspiration for everyone, you may want to choose a profession that provides some of the same rewards researchers found in studying conductors:

• Fulfillment on a very personal level

• A chance for widespread recognition of accomplishment

• An opportunity to channel stress in creative, productive ways

Unfortunately, there's very little data on other occupations that lend themselves to long-life contentment. However, it is known that certain jobs are risky in and of themselves. According to the National Safe Workplace Institute in Chicago, 60,000 to 70,000 people a year die from on-the-job accidents or illnesses caused by working conditions (e.g., exposure to chemicals or other noxious materials). Table 5-3 lists the riskiest industries and some of the occupations within each, based on U.S. Department of Labor statistics.

Incidentally, if you're a woman, the greatest on-the-job mortality risk you're likely to face is murder. That's because women typically don't take high-risk blue-collar jobs like firefighter, but they do take jobs tending the cash register in grocery stores, gas stations and liquor stores—prime targets for robbers who become murderers.

Table 5-3 | The Riskiest Industries

If you're in the market for a new occupation, you might want to know which industries are most likely to cause serious injuries or cut your life short. Below are listed industries and typical occupations within each, in order from riskiest to least risky. The rankings are based on the incidence of deaths, injuries and illnesses reported per 100 full-time workers per year:

Industry	Incidents Per 100 Full-Time Workers Per Year
Construction	14.3
Roofing, siding and sheet-metal work	
Nonresidential building construction (ex.: construction workers and carpenters' helpers)	
Masonry, stonework and plastering	
Plumbing, heating and air conditioning	
Manufacturing	13.1
Ship- and boat-building repair	
Meat processing	
Iron and steel foundry work	
Metal forging and stamping (ex.: metal molders)	
Logging and sawmill work (ex.: timber cutters and loggers)	

(continued)

Table 5-3 | The Riskiest Industries *(continued)*

Industry	Incidents Per 100 Full-Time Workers Per Year
Agriculture, forestry and fishing	10.9
Farming	
Forestry work	
Transportation and public utilities	9.2
Sanitation work (ex.: garbage collectors)	
Air transportation (ex.: airline pilots and flight attendants)	
Truck driving	
Dock work	
Trolley, bus and taxi transportation (ex.: taxi drivers and chauffeurs)	
Mining	8.5
Oil and gas field work	
Coal mining	
Metal mining	
Wholesale and retail trade	8.0
Food sales	
Building-supply sales	

Industry	Incidents Per 100 Full-Time Workers Per Year
Services	5.5
Nursing	
Hotel and motel work	
Hospital work	
Financial, insurance and real estate	2.0
Real estate work	
Insurance-industry work	
Banking	

Source: "BLS Estimates of Occupational Injury and Illness Incidence Rates for Selected Industries, 1989." Bureau of Labor Statistics, U.S. Department of Labor.

6 | Medical Care

I f death from medical miscare were a category sanctioned by compilers of vital statistics, it would rank as Number Three Cause of Death. The estimated 170,000+ medical miscare deaths per year would trail only heart disease (760,000) and cancer (480,000); and they would be comfortably ahead of cerebrovascular diseases (150,000), accidental death (95,000) and pulmonary disease (78,000).

At the same time, a wisely chosen medical practitioner can screen you appropriately for a life-threatening disease and detect it in its early stages, when you have the best chance of cure. He can protect your child from diseases such as polio, which doctors have nearly wiped out in the Western Hemisphere (with worldwide eradication expected by the year 2000). When you are seriously ill or in danger, a good doctor can save your life.

The key phrase to remember is "good doctor." Because, although even the best doctors make mistakes, your chances of survival increase considerably when you're in competent hands. Here's how to take advantage of the best in the medical profession without being victimized by the worst.

59 | Evaluate Your Doctor to See Whether a Change Is in Order

Marcus Welby, M.D., is everyone's idea of the perfect doctor — friendly, caring, skillful, communicative, ready to treat the patient as an equal, even making house calls. There are plenty of Marcus Welbys out there; you just have to find them amidst the doctors who withhold information, are inconsiderate or careless, don't listen, think they're God's gift to mankind, or think they are God themselves.

It's important to get the right doctor because minor health problems mixed with negative doctor traits can become major (and even life-threatening) problems. If you already have a major affliction, you need someone to handle it properly.

You probably already have a family doctor. You may be perfectly satisfied with her – or maybe you just think you are. To evaluate whether your doctor is giving you the kind of care you need to live to 100, ask yourself these 10 important questions:

1. *Does your doctor communicate well?* Communication is a give-and-take business. Your physician should be ready, willing and able to explain your condition and recommended treatments in language and terminology you understand. If you don't get it, it should be explained again. At the same time, a good communicator has the ability to listen, too. The doctor should hear your concerns and questions, indicate they've been heard, then respond appropriately with answers and information. This is especially important for elderly patients, whom doctors frequently regard as their most persnickety customers. Studies have shown that the questions and demands of elderly patients are often downplayed, tuned out or ignored altogether.

2. *Does your doctor give you the bum's rush?* Doctors are businesspeople and they need to make a profit. They do pretty well, too, with the average general practitioner netting an annual income of about $103,000 after business expenses and before taxes. But to accomplish this, many doctors run assembly-line operations, with their nurses doing many of the basic routines not requiring a doctor's training – measuring weight, temperature, blood pressure and so forth. The doctor races in and

out of the room like a Supermarket Sweep game-show contestant blowing through the cereal aisle. Efficiency should not become haste; your doctor should spend as much time as necessary and should not pressure you to cut the visit short in order to tap the next wallet.

3. *Does your doctor discuss treatment alternatives?* There are often many ways to skin a health problem. Clogged arteries can be "fixed" temporarily with bypass surgery, angioplasty or medication and lifestyle changes. Each choice has its pros and cons. Your doctor should be ready to map out your options based on proven efficacy, cost, discomfort and risk.

4. *Does your doctor treat you like an equal?* Too many patients approach their doctors from a subordinate position, placing the physicians high upon a pedestal; unfortunately, many doctors are eager to go along with this script. This can lead to erroneous assumptions that a doctor's word is gospel. Your relationship with your physician should be based on equality and mutual respect. Working with your doctor – instead of just following orders – is crucial because you have a responsibility to participate in and direct your own treatment.

5. *How good a diagnostician is your doctor?* One of the weakest links in the medical-care chain is diagnosis. With the advent of more and more lab tests and high-tech divining rods, diagnosis is becoming a lost art. Your doctor should know an uncomplicated backache from a symptom of kidney disease.

6. *Are you comfortable with your doctor?* This is a gut assessment, but it's an important factor to weigh. Your visits should be pleasant, friendly. You and the doctor should have a rapport. You should not walk out feeling that you have been a bother.

7. *Is your doctor's price right?* Doctor fees are not chiseled in stone—they are negotiable. While this is an important pocketbook issue and a benchmark against which you can assess quality of care, price is also a measure of your doctor's attitude toward patients. A gouger is sending a clear message about the way he balances commitments to the Hippocratic Oath and the profit motive.

8. *Do you trust your doctor?* You have to follow your instincts here, but you shouldn't place your health in the hands of a doctor whose judgment you doubt. The physician you choose should instill trust in you.

9. *Is your doctor a good advocate?* This becomes more crucial the more incapacitated you are, because when you are vulnerable, you need a doctor who looks out for your best interests. A doctor should evidence caring about your needs and interests. In the normal course of a doctor/patient relationship, this caring comes out in her visible concern, familiarity with your health interests, and attempts to keep you from truly unnecessary testing, procedures and expenses.

10. *Is your doctor a believer in preventive medicine?* Doctors who promote improved nutrition, physical fitness and other wellness practices can save you sick time and money. All the better if such doctors also practice what they preach.

If your present doctor doesn't meet these standards, shop around for a new one. Get referrals from friends who are satisfied with their own physicians. Nurses may know the most about the doctors in your area—both the superb physicians and the duds. Use your doctor's day off to check out the covering physician.

You may not need a top-quality doctor for every cough

and cold, but having a real pro who makes the right call at the right time and who knows how to act decisively and correctly in a pinch may mean the difference between life and death for you somewhere down the road.

60 | If You Have Children, Work With Your Doctor To Get Them Immunized On Schedule

Immunizations are one of the great success stories of modern medicine. Doctors have wiped out smallpox and are nearing eradication of polio as well. Yet sometimes we take this miracle for granted. Although the vast majority of children have completed their immunizations by the time they enter kindergarten or first grade (because the laws in most states require it), the Centers for Disease Control says that one-fourth of all preschoolers are not up to date on their immunizations. This leaves millions of kids vulnerable to a host of diseases, from measles to whooping cough. As a result, many childhood diseases that were once near eradication have made a comeback. In 1990 there were 28,000 measles cases, the worst epidemic in 10 years. Whooping cough, which can cause seizures, brain damage and even death, has increased fourfold in 10 years, while rubella (German measles) has tripled.

This is an area where you need to work closely with your doctor to make sure your child is being immunized on time, particularly if your child is in preschool, day care or some other group situation. The American Academy of Pediatrics recommends the schedule set out in Table 6-1. If your doctor suggests a different schedule, ask for his rationale.

Table 6-1 | Your Child's Immunization Schedule

Below is the schedule of immunizations and boosters recommended at different ages by the American Academy of Pediatrics. Immunizations are for Hepatitis B; Diphtheria/Tetanus/Pertussis (whooping cough) (DTP); Polio; Measles/Mumps/Rubella (MMR); Haemophilus Influenzae B (Hib), the strain of bacteria that causes meningitis; and Tetanus/Diphtheria (Td). An MMR booster is recommended at 11 to 12 years, but is given earlier in some locales because of local epidemics. Ages and doses of Hepatitis B vaccine vary, depending on which of several available kinds your child has had and at what age.

Age	Vaccine
Birth	Hepatitis B
1-2 months	Hepatitis B
2 months	DTP, Polio, Haemophilus influenzae B (Hib)
4 months	DTP, Polio, Hib
6 months	DTP, possibly Hib (doses vary)
6-18 months	Hepatitis B
12-15 months	Possibly Hib (doses vary)
15 months	MMR, possibly Hib (doses vary)
15-18 months	DTP, Polio
4-6 years	DTP, Polio
11-12 years	MMR
14-16 years	Td

61 | Keep Track of The Immunizations You'll Need As an Adult—And Get Them When Necessary

Immunization isn't just for kids; it's something you must have to pay attention to periodically throughout life. For instance, every 10 years you should get a booster for tetanus and diphtheria; immunity against these deadly diseases simply wears off with time. It's been well established that elderly people benefit from vaccines against influenza just before flu season, since they're much more likely to suffer serious complications from the bug than the rest of the population.

At the age of 100, Elmer Shuster of Westerville, Ohio, has life by the tail. He doesn't smoke or drink and leans toward a vegetarian diet (though he does eat some poultry). When you ask him why he lived so long, he ponders the fact that he "lived like everybody else, but I worked hard." Indeed, Elmer credits his long life to the exercise and fresh air he got while building houses most of his adult life.

What about those mainstays of modern health, doctors and drugs? "Well, I didn't use them much," he admits. "All I ever took were pills for circulation." Elmer stays connected to the life around him; he's interested in world politics and reads voraciously. Though he's down to earth, he's not—as he puts it—a "homebody."

Interestingly, research has found that elderly patients are more likely to contract pneumonia if they have had hospital care within the past four years. According to a *Journal of the American Medical Association* report of a study of Medicare beneficiaries discharged with medical diagnoses of pneumonia, a whopping 62 percent of those people had been in a hospital at least once within the previous four years, and not necessarily for pneumonia. Eighty-seven percent of those pneumonia patients had some sort of high-risk condition, such as heart disease or diabetes. In light of this and another important study showing that hospital care is a marker for identifying people at increased risk for hospital admission and death from pneumonia, experts recommend that elderly hospital patients consider a pneumonia vaccine when they leave the hospital.

62 | Look Over Your Doctor's Shoulder for Misdiagnosis

Even a good GP, of course, has limits, and in many cases she knows them. But too frequently, she may diagnose or just not see a problem that is actually there. Often these errors occur because of defects in the doctor/patient relationship, which is why carefully choosing your doctor is so important.

According to Joel Dimsdale, M.D., of the psychiatry department of Massachusetts General Hospital, in Boston, diagnostic dissonance can occur in a doctor when the patient comes from a group (racial, professional, economic or other) with which the doctor is uncomfortable; when the patient's behavior makes the doctor uncomfortable or angry; when the patient is too close to the doctor, as with a relative or colleague; or when the doctor is uncomfortable with the patient's illness.

Misdiagnosis and oversight can also result from the fact that so many diseases and conditions share many of the same symptoms. AIDS, for example, can present itself in a variety of ways that don't leap out at the doctor. Clinical depression is a classic strikeout situation for GPs. Family doctors, who are untrained in detecting major depressive disorders, diagnose this problem correctly less than half the time. Often, doctors' preconceived notions—about women or the elderly, for example—cause them to dismiss the symptoms of depression as simply the blues or the onset of senility and old age.

But doctors can also miss loud and clear warning signs of serious trouble. Aside from spontaneous human combustion, symptoms don't scream out much louder than those related to heart attack. But in a study by E.J. Zarling, M.D., and colleagues of 100 autopsies on people who had conclusively died of heart failure, researchers looked back at how attending physicians diagnosed the situation before death. Myocardial infarction was not spotted in a shocking 47 percent of cases! Worse, in half the incorrect diagnoses, the doctor was a cardiologist.

Knowing that doctors are capable of making mistakes gets you halfway to a solution; you won't blindly follow their every prescription. But you've also got to take further action on your own. If you think your doctor's off track, insist on resolving your suspicions. Research the symptoms in your family medical guide and at a library. Don't let the doctor tell you you're just paranoid about cancer or some other dread disease; trust your own instincts. Be ready to veto the prescriptions if you're not satisfied.

And perhaps the most important remedy of all: Seek specialists when you have more difficult problems. Reason: Because of their narrower focus on a specific group of disorders, specialists have more experience diagnosing those diseases. A cancer specialist, say, sees many more cases of the disease than your GP, who might encounter only two new cases of cancer per year. So a specialist should more easily see the obvious signs, better sense the hidden nuances, unmask misleading symptoms and arrive at a more accurate diagnosis.

As with all else in the inexact art and science of medicine, however, even specialists are not infallible and bear watching. Just ask those cardiologists who failed to recognize the heart attacks mentioned earlier.

63 | Go Right to the Top Specialist For a Second Opinion

When should you seek a second opinion?

1) When you have an especially complex, confounding or chronic medical problem

2) Before any serious treatments, such as surgery, chemo-therapy or radiation therapy

3) After any foreboding medical verdicts involving the status "terminal," "incurable" or "low survivability"

4) When the prescribed treatments and remedies are not working

You can see a nearby specialist, but when you are dealing with a serious or potentially fatal condition, there are definite advantages to going right to the top in the field.

In general, top doctors are associated with major academic medical centers. This combination provides physicians who have greater experience with tough cases because they deal with large regional and national patient pools. They're also backed by technological resources and staff, state-of-the-art treatments and procedures, and higher levels of diagnostic intuition and sophistication that most local specialists just can't bring to the case.

To find these marvels of medicine, ask your doctor. Any medical practitioner worth his salt should be able to direct you to the top medical centers and some of the top-name specialists in your region or the nation who cover the suspected disorder. From time to time major city and national magazines, such as *New York* magazine, *Philadelphia* magazine, *Washingtonian*, *Prevention* magazine and *U.S. News & World Report*, run listings of top medical centers and specialists. Hang onto these reference guides.

We asked specialists and medical experts around the United States to recommend the leading hospitals for a variety of specialties in serious diseases and complex conditions. The results appear in Table 6-2. This list is by no means all-inclusive, but it can provide a good lead to some of the best care in the nation.

Once you locate a medical mecca, don't check your normal consumerist wits at the admissions desk. Be mindful of the fact that specialists have a tendency to filter your problem through their area of expertise. So a neurologist may attribute your severe headaches to a brain disorder when the actual cause may be too much coffee.

And even the best specialists make mistakes. Take the case of Dr. C. Everett Koop's eye problem.

The U.S. Surgeon General was rushing to an appointment in Iowa when he began seeing double. Dr. Thomas Weingeist, head of ophthalmology at the University of Iowa Hospitals and

Clinics in Iowa City, gave Koop the once over. The problem had resurfaced from time to time ever since Koop suffered a football injury to the head some 50 years earlier.

"He didn't have much time in his schedule, so I referred him to a superstar in the Washington area," recalls Weingeist. Koop visited that doctor in the capital, then phoned Weingeist.

"He recommended surgery," said Koop. "What do you think?"

"I think you should get a second opinion," answered Weingeist, who gave his 68-year-old patient the name of another D.C. superdoc.

That doctor found a very simple, nonsurgical solution: Koop needed new eyeglasses.

The point for those who would live 100 years: All surgery is a risk—approximately 1.3 percent of all people undergoing operations die. If a second opinion can preclude taking that risk, it's time and money well spent.

At 100, Fannie Reed says the secret to a long life is work. "I've always worked hard," she says. But she also seems to have added years to her life by taking the lead with her own medical care. She's always had good relationships with her doctors and never takes medicine—"except Bufferin to help with pain," she interjects. Perhaps her wisest life-preserving medical philosophy has to do with hospitals and the several operations she's had. "When I've been in the hospital, I wanted to get out as fast as possible. I just don't like them," she adds.

Table 6-2 | Top Medical Centers

The alphabetical listing below shows some of the leading hospitals in the medical specialties indicated, as recommended by specialists and experts in those fields.

Specialty	Leading Medical Centers
Cancer	Dana-Farber Cancer Institute, Boston
	Fred Hutchinson Cancer Research Center, Seattle
	Georgetown University Vince Lombardi Cancer Research Center, Washington, DC
	Johns Hopkins University Hospital, Baltimore
	Mayo Clinic, Rochester, Minn.
	M.D. Anderson Cancer Center, Houston
	Memorial Sloan-Kettering Cancer Center, New York
	University of Pittsburgh Medical Center, Pittsburgh
Cardiology	Barnes Hospital, St. Louis
	Baylor Hospitals, Dallas
	Brigham and Women's Hospital, Boston
	Cedar's Sinai Hospital UCLA, Los Angeles
	Cleveland Clinic, Cleveland
	Columbia-Presbyterian Hospital, New York
	Duke University Hospital, Durham, N.C.
	Emory University Hospital, Atlanta

Specialty	Leading Medical Centers
Cardiology *(continued)*	Massachusetts General Hospital, Boston,
	Mayo Clinic, Rochester, Minn.
	Mid-America Heart Institute, Kansas City, Mo.
	Stanford University Hospital, Palo Alto, Calif.
	Texas Heart Institute, Houston
	Yale-New Haven Medical Center, New Haven, Conn.
Endocrinology	Cleveland Clinic, Cleveland
	Jackson Memorial (University of Miami) Hospital, Miami
	Jewish Hospital, St. Louis
	Massachusetts General Hospital, Boston
	Mayo Clinic, Rochester, Minn.
	Stanford University Hospital, Palo Alto, Calif.
	UCLA Medical Center, Los Angeles
Gastroenterology	Johns Hopkins University Hospital, Baltimore
	Massachusetts General Hospital, Boston
	Mayo Clinic, Rochester, Minn.
	Mt. Sinai Hospital, New York
	University of Chicago Hospitals, Chicago
	University of Pittsburgh Medical Center, Pittsburgh

(continued)

Table 6-2 | **Top Medical Centers** (*continued*)

Specialty	Leading Medical Centers
Neurology	Hospital of the University of Pennsylvania, Philadelphia
	Johns Hopkins University Hospital, Baltimore
	Massachusetts General Hospital, Boston
	Mayo Clinic, Rochester, Minn.
	Tufts New England Medical Center, Boston
	UCLA Medical Center, Los Angeles
	University of California San Francisco Medical Center, San Francisco
Obstetrics/ Gynecology	Georgetown University Medical Center, Washington, DC
	Jones Institute for Reproductive Medicine, Norfolk, Va.
	Northwestern Memorial Hospital, Chicago
	Ohio State University Hospital, Columbus, Ohio
	St. Barnabas Medical Center, Livingston, N.J.
	University of California at Irvine Medical Center, Irvine, Calif.
	University of California at San Diego Medical Center, San Diego
	University of Kansas Medical Center, Kansas City, Mo.
	University of Southern California Medical Center, Los Angeles

Specialty	Leading Medical Centers
Psychiatry	Columbia-Presbyterian Hospital, New York
	Dartmouth Hitchcock Medical Center, Lebanon, N.H.
	McLean Hospital, Belmont, Mass.
	North Carolina Memorial Hospital, Chapel Hill, N.C.
	Payne Whitney Clinic, New York
	Southwestern Medical Center, Dallas
	UCLA Medical Center, Los Angeles
	University of Washington Medical Center, Seattle

64 | If You're a Woman, Get A Baseline Mammogram At Age 35—With More Mammograms Every Two To Three Years Afterward (Annually After Age 50)

Breast cancer is the most common form of cancer among women; 1 in 10 will get it in her lifetime. Most deaths from breast cancer are preventable if the disease is detected early, and mammograms are part of the early screening process. Mammograms enable doctors to detect tumors before they're large enough to feel–giving your doctor (and you) a fighting chance of beating the disease. You should pay particular attention to mammograms if you have a history of breast cancer in your family (for more information on finding this out, see Chapter 3), or if you are undergoing estrogen replacement therapy (ERT) to help fend off heart disease after menopause. Both these situations greatly increase your risk of getting breast cancer.

You should also ask your medical practitioner to teach you the proper technique for monthly breast self-examinations. Since mammograms are not infallible, it's good to have another early-warning signal to fall back on.

65 | Avoid the Hospital Unless Absolutely Necessary— And Stay Only As Long As Necessary

Each year some 2 million hospital patients acquire a nosocomial (hospital-originated) infection; an estimated 100,000 die from these illnesses. Because of the congregation of sickness, hospitals are teeming with infection. You can't mop down the whole hospital with disinfectants or drive yourself crazy doing sentry duty trying to close off every avenue by which these invisible attackers can get you.

But you can take some important precautions. The best way to avoid nosocomial infection is to avoid the hospital. One way to do that is to opt for outpatient procedures, if possible. If you are hospitalized, the shorter your stay, the better.

Technological advances in surgery have made it possible

for 51 percent of all surgery to be handled on an outpatient basis. Outpatient surgery can be accomplished at the hospital's outpatient unit, in your specialist's office or at a freestanding ambulatory surgical center not associated with a hospital.

66 | If You Need Surgery, Choose the Least Invasive Techniques Available

Few things are more inviting of infection than a large surgical gash. Surgical advances now allow many procedures to be accomplished with a tiny incision; the surgeon "gets inside" you with fiber-optic video equipment and catheter-controlled surgical equipment. Other avenues to explore with specialists include laser surgery and ultrasonography.

67 | If You Must Stay in A Hospital, Insist That Any Medical Professional Who Comes in Contact With You Simply Wash Her Hands First

Doctors and nurses don't do enough of this–despite the rec-ommendations of the Centers for Disease Control and the American Hospital Association–and infection can easily hitchhike a ride from the last infected patient or surface onto the health-care professional's hands and onto you.

68 | Limit the Use of Urinary Catheters

Urinary-tract infections account for 42 percent of all noso-comial infections, and catheters provide a good highway for bacteria into a very susceptible breeding ground. Urinary-tract infections acquired during catheterization have been associated with a threefold increase in mortality among hospital patients. Experts say catheters are often misused and left in longer than necessary. As long as a catheter is in, ask nurses to regularly check the catheter's drainage and help you keep clean. And ask doctors and nurses to get that tube out ASAP. Also ask that chemical depilatories be used for presurgery hair removal. One study indicates that hair removal by depilatory instead of razor reduces infection rates by 90 percent.

69 | Find Out If Your Hospital Roommate Puts You at Risk Of Infection Through Shared Bathroom Facilities or Airborne Transmission

If so, ask to be transferred to another room. This doesn't make you a troublemaker. You have a right to protect your health from identifiable risk sources. And if a nosocomial infection keeps you in the hospital longer than necessary, who do you think the hospital is going to send the extra billing charges to—your roommate, the hospital gratis services office or you?

70 | If You're a Man Aged 40 Or More, Get a Prostate Exam Once a Year

The prostate, a walnut-size gland that helps produce the fluid in semen, is the second most likely site of cancer among men (after the lungs). In the early stages, there are often no symptoms, which is why a yearly screening procedure is needed. The most common method of diagnosis involves a digital rectal exam, but doctors have also come up with a new blood-screening test, called PSA, to help in early detection. Ask your doctor about this screening procedure. A rectal and colon exam should begin yearly at this age, too.

71 | Get an Advocate When Hospitalized

When you are incapacitated in a hospital, you are vulnerable to the mistakes and blunders of dozens of strangers—doctors, nurses, pharmacists, food-service personnel, candy stripers, interns, technicians, housekeepers, other employees and visitors. Medical equipment can malfunction. Tests can be misinterpreted. Files and records can be mixed up. An estimated 22,000 to 36,000 doctors in practice are alcoholics, recovering alcoholics or wannabe alcoholics. And approximately 100,000 employed nurses suffer from drug or alcohol dependence, according to the American Nursing Association's Committee on Impaired Nursing Practices.

The best way to protect yourself is to be vigilant for errors, ask questions about anything you don't understand, and unabashedly stand up for immediate corrections. Why has your medication, its dosage or its frequency suddenly changed? If you're supposed to be getting a CAT scan, why are you being transported to pre-op? If your name is Mary Smith, why were Maureen Jones' flowers delivered to you; has your identification been mistakenly switched?

Sometimes you are physically unable to watch out for your own interests (because of sedation, unconsciousness, disorientation), your judgment is impaired or you just can't get the attention of the powers that be. In that case, you need others – maybe several others – to act as your advocates.

Your doctor is a good person to have on your team, by virtue of his authority and your relationship. Befriend members of the nursing staff, who have a different kind of power – de facto authority. Enlist your spouse, friends, offspring or relatives to look out for your interests as well. Many hospitals also have patient representatives or ombudsmen who offer varying degrees of effectiveness.

Whomever you choose, make sure your advocates are assertive, intelligent and ready to stand firm should the hospital challenge their authority to act on your behalf.

72 | If You're a Woman Aged 18 Or More, Get a Yearly Pap Smear and Pelvic Exam— Unless There Have Been Three Consecutive Negative Results; Then You Can Be Tested Every Three Years

Pap smears and pelvic exams have cut dramatically the incidence of cervical cancer in the United States, because they help detect cell changes in the cervix at a very early stage. If a teenager is sexually active before the age of 18, she, too, should have Pap smears and pelvic exams, because early sexual activity is a risk factor.

73 | Beware the Sandman

An estimated 10,000 deaths per year occur because of mistakes in administering anesthesia. Of course, the actual incidence of deaths wholly or partially attributable to anesthesia is low in comparison to the number of operations performed—between 1 and 2.5 deaths per 10,000 anesthesia patients. But the risk is significant enough to warrant safeguarding yourself. Once you've gone under, you can't keep an eye on the anesthesiologist, so you've got to find out beforehand (from your doctor) who your anesthesiologist is and hunt her down. Ask the anesthesiologist to meet with you sometime during the day before your operation. A last-minute, late-night visit isn't good enough; insist on a daytime consultation when you are alert and still have time to make changes.

The anesthesiologist should have questions for you about potential trouble spots that can put you to sleep permanently: heart problems, allergies, high or low blood pressure, adverse reactions to past anesthesia and more.

You should have questions for the anesthesiologist, too. What kind of anesthesia will be used? Why? What are the risk factors? Does she have any particular concerns about your case? What sort of pre-op procedures should you follow (such as what time should you cease eating or taking liquids)? What should you expect in the operating room and in recovery? Will the anesthesiologist be present in the operating room or will an intern, nurse anesthetist or some other substitute do the actual sedating? The highly paid anesthesiologist should be doing the actual hands-on work for you, so insist that you get what you're paying for and get an agreement in writing requiring her to perform the work.

You should also use your meeting as an opportunity to size up the anesthesiologist. Does she seem reliable, competent, level-headed? If you have doubts, get someone else.

74 | Be Cautious With Prescription Drugs

Inside and outside the hospital, always thoroughly understand your pharmaceutical prescriptions, because mistakes always can be and are made. What kind of mistakes? Wrong dosages, adverse reactions, wrong kind of medication for the problem, drug interactions (particularly for elderly patients who may be on several medications) and undesirable side effects are just some of the possibilities. Often the amount of drug prescribed is wrong for a patient's weight, or there are multiple prescriptions being filled at several different pharmacies, with nobody to oversee their safety in combination. Overmedication and the potential for addiction to painkillers are yet other dangers. Any one of these negatives can lead to death.

To protect yourself, whenever your doctor prescribes medication, have him answer four questions:

1) What benefits will this medication provide?

2) What negative side effects can I expect?

3) These are the other drugs I am currently taking. Will there be any bad drug interactions?

4) How soon can I stop taking this medication?

Double-check your doctor's advice with your pharmacist.

75 | Practice Preventive Medicine

The best way by far to protect yourself against harm by the medical profession is to sidestep the need for medical care by adopting a healthier lifestyle. A lifelong healthy lifestyle is important enough in your younger years, but it is absolutely critical for the benefits it can bring to your older years.

"Through practice of appropriate life skills, you minimize the risk and degree of future chronic ailments and can better manage existing ones," says George Pfeiffer, a leading health expert at the Center for Corporate Health Promotion in Reston, Virginia. Among such good life skills: staying active and involved with life, managing stress, eating healthfully, using alcohol in moderation, staying physically fit, not smoking and avoiding accidents.

A lifetime of poor health practices can lead to chronic ailments, debilitation and isolation in your later years. That is the first step on a slippery slope ending in premature death before age 100. So, as the philosophy behind this book emphasizes, the best approach is to avoid the avoidable whenever possible.

7 | Sound Body

Most of the advice in this book so far has centered on what you should do to your body to keep it running smoothly for 100 years (at least)—what nutrients you should put into it, what exercise paces you should put it through to keep it in prime condition, what dangerous environments you should keep it out of, and what doctors can do to help (or hurt) your body.

Now it's time to shift perspective and look at the marvelous machine itself. Here's how to keep a scorecard on where you've been and where you're going. And if you don't like what you see before you, maybe it's time to set a new course.

76 | If You Smoke, Make Quitting The Top Priority in Your Life

It's more important than getting that new promotion, it's more important than driving the kids to Little League games, it's even more important than a good sex life. You can follow every other long-life prescription in this book, but if you also smoke, you risk undoing it all. Smoking is so hard on the body that it affects multiple organs and systems and puts you at risk for a great deal more than lung cancer. Here's a selected list of diverse effects smoking has on the body, based on a variety of studies around the world:

•Most women don't have heart attacks until after menopause, when they lose the protective edge of high estrogen levels. But smoking can help remove the natural protection of youth; researchers say it causes 65 percent of premenopausal heart attacks.

•Smokers who undergo surgery suffer more scarring and heal more slowly than nonsmokers. That's because nicotine constricts the arteries and limits the flow of nourishing blood to skin wounds.

•Smoking reduces the rigidity and duration of men's erections during sex—again, because it constricts arteries and limits blood flow.

•Cigarette smoking helps tear little holes in the linings of the heart and lungs.

•Young women who smoke have spines with decreased bone-mineral density—a condition that puts them at higher risk for crippling osteoporosis later in life.

•Heavy smoking raises blood pressure, a major factor in heart disease, stroke and kidney disease.

You may feel you can't bring yourself to quit just yet, but statistics show you probably will eventually. Younger smokers, those between the ages of 18 and 34, quit at a rate of only about 32 percent, according to the Centers for Disease Control. But by the time they reach the ripe old age of 55 and beyond, the quit rate more than doubles, to 65 percent—proving that you learn a thing or two from youth to middle age.

You may have also heard about the horrors of nicotine withdrawal. But there's another side to the story of what happens physically when you quit: Your body experiences immediate and far-reaching beneficial effects. According to the Chicago Lung Association, within 20 minutes after your final cigarette, your blood pressure and pulse rate drop to normal. Within 24 hours, your chances of a heart attack begin to decrease. In 72 hours, your bronchial tubes relax and your lung capacity increases, making breathing easier. Within 5 to 10 years, your heart and circulatory system have repaired the damage from your smoking habit. And within 10 years, pre-cancerous cells have been replaced. The lung-cancer death rate decreases to nearly that of a nonsmoker.

Still think you can't do it? You may need the help of a support group. For information about a Nicotine Anonymous group in your area, write to Nicotine Anonymous World Services, 2118 Greenwich Street, San Francisco, CA 94123.

When Alabamian Nelson Shears was born on March 8, 1885, the United States was still very much an agrarian society, with some 42 percent of the population living on farms (vs. a scant 2 percent today). The 107-year-old Nelson says working the land may have been responsible for giving him so many years. "I've been a farmer all my life," he says. Nelson started farming for a living in 1908, at age 20, first as a sharecropper and later with his own land in Browns Station, Alabama. "I've raised cotton, corn and hogs," he says.

Now a resident of Selma, Nelson can still be seen out tilling the soil with his hoe, "planting peas and some little butter beans" whose wholesome goodness you can almost taste. What makes farming a fountain of youth? "Doing hard work outdoors in the fields, breathing the fresh air and staying active are good for you," he explains. Nelson says there are only two more things folks need to remember if they want to live a long life: "Stay out of bad company and don't drink whiskey or beer."

77 | Never Diet Again

You heard us—never diet again. Yes, extra pounds—particularly around the abdomen—present a greatly increased risk of diabetes, heart disease, stroke and even cancer—four of the top killers in America. Some 15 percent of women and 10 percent of men are obese, which means that they exceed their ideal weight by at least 20 percent. Many, many more people carry some extra pounds that are straining their hearts as well as their seams. And the vast majority of Americans have been on at least one weight-loss diet in their lifetimes, but where has it gotten them?

Though millions of individuals are able to lose dozens (and sometimes hundreds) of pounds, 90 percent of them gain it all back, often with a little something extra the second, third or fourth time around. This is not necessarily the fault of the diets themselves, though there are some wacky fad diets of questionable safety (and effectiveness). It is the fault of the dieting concept.

As harmful as obesity is, we now know that the up-and-down, gain-and-lose pattern known as *yo-yo dieting* is worse. Yo-yo dieting confuses the body's weight-regulation system so badly that each diet makes it harder to lose weight the next time. Then, too, gaining and losing weight repeatedly appears to strongly increase heart risk. The well-known Framingham Heart Study, which has monitored thousands of people for 40 years, showed that overweight people who shed 10 percent of their body weight decreased their coronary risk by 20 percent. But if they gained the weight back, they added a 30 percent risk to their lives—leaving them worse off than when they had started. Imagine the effects of doing this repeatedly throughout a lifetime.

So what's the answer—to sigh and accept the health risk of extra pounds? Not really. But as long as you focus on pounds and dieting (which to many people feels like "deprivation"), you are likely to lose and regain, lose and regain, over and over. A better idea is to throw away your scale and focus on developing a healthful, lifelong eating plan—not a temporary diet—based on the low-fat nutritional concepts presented in Chapter 1 and a sensible exercise plan based on the concepts in Chapter 2. When you're not looking, the pounds will slowly—and permanently—come off.

There's an old saying that happiness is a by-product. So it is with permanent weight loss; the more you pursue it as an obsessive goal, the more elusive it becomes. When you forget about it and concentrate on healthful body choices, reasonable weight is the inevitable by-product.

78 | Keep Your Blood Pressure Low Through Natural Means, Such As Maintaining A Reasonable Weight And Exercising

High blood pressure has been called the silent killer, and with good reason. An estimated 60 million Americans have it; nearly half of those don't have any idea that they do. Untreated, high blood pressure, or *hypertension,* can lead to stroke, heart attack or kidney failure—and take 15 years off your life.

Mary's Massmann's advice: Don't drink or smoke. "Those two things can hurt you more than anything else," she says. And *do* eat right.

Mary says her other secret to long life is friends, particularly her close 50-year friendship with her compatriot Jan. "That probably helped a lot," says 100-year-old Mary. "I could talk to her when I had problems, she always made me feel better. She was a real, true friend." Mary met her special friend when Jan's husband got his jacket zipper stuck at a social gathering. "I had a pair of pliers in my pocketbook," Mary laughs. "It worked."

How do you tell whether you're part of this club no one wants to belong to? For most people, there are no clear-cut symptoms to push them toward a doctor's office. If there are any signs at all, they're the kind that could be mistaken for anything: a headache in the back of the head or upper neck, particularly first thing in the morning; perhaps some dizziness or light-headedness when going from a sitting to standing position; maybe some heart palpitations. That's why yearly monitoring of blood pressure is so important.

There are many ways to reduce high blood pressure, including giving up smoking, increasing exercise, cutting back on salt, losing weight and taking an antihypertensive drug. Your doctor may recommend some combination of these approaches, but the one thing you want to avoid is relying purely on a drug to cure the problem. A lifetime of healthy living is far more likely to get you to the ripe old age of 100 than a lifetime of compensatory drugs.

The exact threshold for a diagnosis of hypertension has changed in recent years, and is still a matter of contention among some doctors. Table 7-1 lists the most commonly accepted ranges for both normal and hypertensive patients, based on a report from the National Institutes of Health.

79 | Get a Full Lipoprotein Analysis—And If Your Cholesterol Levels Are High, Take Steps to Lower Them

Lots of people know that their total cholesterol count should be lower than 200. Between 200 and 240 is considered "borderline high," and 240 or more is a definite signal for medical intervention. But total cholesterol count is not necessarily the total picture. Many doctors feel a truer indicator of cholesterol health is the ratio of high-density lipoprotein, or HDL (the good cholesterol), to overall cholesterol.

HDL is "good" cholesterol because it keeps low-density lipoprotein, or LDL (the "bad" cholesterol) from depositing itself in arteries. These LDL deposits help fatty plaques develop on arterial walls, leading to atherosclerosis. When narrowed, clogged arteries interrupt normal blood flow to the heart and brain, the result is a heart attack or stroke.

To keep you safe, your HDL should be above 45 if you're a man and 55 if you're a woman, according to cholesterol expert and Aerobics Center founder Kenneth Cooper, M.D. The American Heart Association also says that an LDL level of 130 to 159 is "borderline high," and LDL of 160 or more is high risk.

Table 7-1 | How Do Your Numbers Stack Up?

If you're in a high-risk group, you should pay particular attention to your blood-pressure numbers, which will most likely increase as you get older. Those in a high-risk group are African-American, obese, have a family history of high blood pressure or are taking birth-control pills. The systolic (top) number measures the pressure when your heart contracts to pump blood; the diastolic (bottom) number measures the pressure when your heart is waiting to pump again. Because you can get vastly different readings depending on who is taking your pressure, it's best to get two separate readings on two different occasions before deciding whether you have high blood pressure.

Blood Pressure (mmHg)	Category
Systolic	
Less than 140	Normal
140-159	Borderline
160 or more	Hypertension
Diastolic	
Less than 85	Normal
85-89	High Normal
90-104	Mild Hypertension
105-114	Moderate Hypertension
115 or more	Severe Hypertension

Source: "The 1988 Report of the Joint National Committee on Detection, Evaluation and Treatment of High Blood Pressure," National Institutes of Health.

Cooper says 75 percent of those with an abnormal lipid profile (high total cholesterol or LDL; or low HDL) can improve that profile by losing weight, starting an exercise program and following five dietary guidelines: (1) reducing total fat intake to 30 percent; (2) reducing saturated fat to 10 percent; (3) increasing the proportion of monounsaturated fats in the diet; (4) reducing dietary cholesterol to 300 mg. a day; and (5) increasing soluble fiber. Each of these strategies is discussed in Chapter 1.

For the remaining 25 percent of patients, medication may be necessary. Luckily, newly developed anticholesterol medications like lovastatin and cholestipol are able to not only reduce cholesterol in the blood, but even reverse the atherosclerotic process once it's begun—providing you keep to a low-fat diet and exercise moderately.

80 | If You Have a Teen Or Preteen at home, Talk Seriously About AIDS

We assume that if you're interested enough in long life to read this book, you know better than to shoot drugs, or have sex without the protection of a condom (unless you're in a long-standing, mutually monogamous relationship). But your kids are another matter. The CDC says 40 percent of ninth graders and 70 percent of twelfth graders have had sex, and half the time they were unprotected by condoms. For that reason, the incidence of AIDS is growing faster among teenagers and young adults than in any other age-group.

Young girls are especially susceptible to infection, since their cervical linings are thinner and more vulnerable to tears during sex. The tears offer a place for human immuno-deficiency virus (HIV), the virus that causes AIDS, to enter the body.

Your own moral code may suggest that teens should be completely abstinent from sex, but you should consider the possibility that your child may look at things differently. If total abstinence is not realistic, recognize that the biggest stumbling block in getting kids to use condoms is the awkwardness of introducing the topic in a moment of passion. You may have to help your teen brainstorm ways to handle this delicate subject. You may also want to suggest ways of exploring sexuality that do not involve intercourse, including massage and masturbation.

One of the best ways to educate kids about AIDS is to get them involved in educating or helping others. Help them find volunteer opportunities with AIDS information hotlines or AIDS victims. Life in the '90s is definitely not "The Waltons," but the kids who survive are likely to be the ones who are realistically prepared.

81 | Drink at Least 8 to 10 8-Oz. Glasses of Water Every Day

Anyone who has ever been to a meeting of a weight-loss support group knows that the biggest complaint is generally not "I'm hungry," but rather "How am I going to drink all that water?" Every responsible weight control approach insists on eight or more glasses of water a day. But we've lost the fine art of drinking something as simple as a glass of water. We drink soda, coffee, iced tea, milk, juice, lemonade—everything but water. It's a national mistake that's unnecessarily costly, in more ways than one.

Our bodies are between 60 and 70 percent water. Water removes toxins from the body through the kidneys, carries nutrients and oxygen to the body in the blood, moistens our lungs to help us breathe, lubricates joints and muscles, and helps our bodies metabolize fat. If you're not drinking enough water, your body may actually retain fluids to protect itself from dehydration—so more water, not less, may be called for when you're retaining fluids.

If you find it impossible to drink eight glasses of water a day to keep your body running with optimal efficiency, try keeping a pitcher of water handy on your desk at work, or nearby as you cook. Occasional sips can add up by the end of the day. You may have to start out with fewer than eight glasses until you get used to the higher volume, but you can increase the amount gradually until you reach your daily goal.

82 | Figure Out How Much Sleep Your Body Needs—And See That You Get It Every Night

Despite the fact that we pamper ourselves in dozens of ways, there's one way in which Americans shortchange themselves repeatedly—in getting adequate sleep. Experts estimate that the vast majority of Americans cheat themselves of one to two hours of needed sleep virtually every night. Reasons are as diverse as the population:

• Twenty-two percent of all employees work at night or on rotating shifts that require them to alternate between day and night work. Because the body has difficulty adjusting to day-time sleep, and particularly to changes back and forth, people in such jobs tend to get less sleep than they need.

• Frequent business travelers have to cope with sleep patterns disrupted by traveling across time zones and by jet lag.

• The availability of late-night television lures millions to stay up past their bedtimes.

• Many of us lead such pressured, hectic lives that we try to squeeze in too many commitments for one 24-hour period — and the place where we compromise is sleep.

Not surprisingly, the number-one complaint doctors hear in their offices is "chronic fatigue." Fatigue impairs judgment and self-control, making us more prone to auto and industrial accidents that cut life short. It also robs us psychologically, making it harder for us to relax or experience pleasure — two important mental attitudes for living to 100.

Studies show that this great American sleep deprivation cuts across age-groups. The National Institute on Aging found that half of all people over the age of 65 often sleep badly and feel poorly rested in the morning. Meanwhile, a Stanford University study of several hundred college or graduate students ages 18 to 30 showed that 20 percent were so chronically underrested, they could fall asleep instantly when asked to lie down in a darkened room.

How do you know whether you're getting enough sleep? Infants generally sleep 16 hours out of every 24, but by the time they're 3, most kids are down to 12 hours a day. From age 6 through adolescence, sleep tends to take up about 10 hours a day. Most adults 18 and over require between 7 and 9 hours of sleep a night; if you're feeling alert and rested when you wake, you're probably in good shape. But here are some trouble signs that indicate your body may be running on empty:

•Inability to get up in the morning without an alarm clock (and sometimes with it)

•Nodding off easily during the day, particularly when doing something tedious

•Constantly low level of energy and general sense of "dragginess"

If you experience these symptoms, experts say you should try going to bed 30 to 90 minutes earlier each night. (Sleeping later the next morning doesn't work as well.) If you also snore heavily during sleep, you may be suffering from sleep apnea, a condition where blocked breathing passages briefly awaken you hundreds of times a night, disturbing the important sleep patterns that help you feel rested and psychologically restored. One study has even linked sleep apnea to increased incidence of high blood pressure. The National Heart, Lung and Blood Institute estimates that 4 percent of the population suffers from this sleep-disturbing disorder.

Another 15 percent of the population is trying desperately to get a decent night's sleep but can't because they have insomnia. Insomnia can be caused by everything from free-floating anxiety to overstimulation by caffeine. If you suffer from this condition, do not take sleeping pills, even if your doctor suggests them. Sleeping pills may literally put you to sleep, but the sleep they provide does not contain the same natural, restful stages as normal sleep—and the pills can be addictive to boot.

If you have a sleep problem that's affecting your health and feelings of well-being, ask your doctor to refer you to a reputable sleep-disorders clinic. As sleep problems become more prevalent, so do such clinics. For more information, write to the American Sleep Disorders Association, 604 Second Street S.W., Rochester, MN 55902.

E.G. of Richmond, Virginia, has spent her 104 years living a life of service and hard work. As a child of a poor farmer, she couldn't go to school because she was needed to take care of younger brothers and sisters. When she grew up, she earned her living as a cook and a maid.

"Working hard helps you to live long," she says. "Working hard, trying to be honest and loving people — that's the biggest thing. Love is like a medicine."

Through E.G.'s humility and honesty shines a strong faith in a power greater than herself. "I got through everything because God was good to me," she says. "I took things as they came because I had faith in Him."

83 | If You Drink Alcohol, Do It Moderately

You've seen the screaming headlines: Red Wine Saves the French From Dying of Heart Attacks! Eat All the Butter, Cream and Roast Duck You Want—As Long As You Wash Them Down with Red Wine! Unfortunately, life is not that simple. Many reasons have been offered to explain why the French are able to eat a high-fat diet without incurring the same risk of heart disease as Americans—including the fact that they eat more fruits, vegetables and fibers, with heart-protecting vitamins and nutrients.

Yet more than one study has concluded that Granny may have known what she was doing when she sipped that one "medicinal" glass of wine or sherry at the end of the day. A large-scale study at Harvard Medical School tracked the health habits of more than 50,000 men, adjusting the data for other coronary risk factors like high blood pressure. It showed conclusively that men who consume alcohol in moderation reduce their risk of heart disease significantly, since a glass of wine a day raises HDL, or "good," cholesterol in the blood and helps protect against atherosclerosis.

Nevertheless, all studies are not that clear on the beneficial effects of alcohol, so moderation is key—particularly if you're overweight. For instance, another study, at the University of Zurich, showed that consumption of alcohol, particularly in high quantities, causes the body to burn fat more slowly than normal. So while a small glass of wine with your evening meal may help your body along to its 100-year mark, a steady diet of three-martini lunches or a six-pack of beer a day will probably lead to a beer gut—and take years off your life.

84 | Protect Yourself Against Ticks and the Diseases They Can Cause

Lyme disease (a condition related to arthritis and caused by a microorganism transmitted through tick bites) has become epidemic throughout the United States, particularly in the Northeast. Because it's difficult to diagnose (it's frequently misdiagnosed as simple arthritis), it often goes undetected and untreated for months, which can result in neurological problems, chronic arthritis, even damage to the heart. In certain parts of the country, ticks also contribute to Rocky Mountain spotted fever, a disease that can be fatal if left untreated.

If you or your children are spending time in a wooded area where ticks are likely to be found, here are some of the precautions you should take to protect yourself:

• Cover as many bare areas of your body as you can. Tuck pants legs into socks and shirttails into pants.

• Wear light-colored clothing that enables you to see ticks more easily.

• Use insect repellent (but doctors don't recommend those containing the chemical DEET for young children, at least on bare skin).

• When you return home, check yourself and your child for ticks, particularly around the hairline. If you find any, remove them with tweezers, grasping the tick as close to the skin as possible. Don't use petroleum jelly, and avoid twisting the tick's head, since it may release infected fluids into the bite. Apply an antiseptic to the site immediately.

• If you have pets who roam outdoors, check them frequently for ticks.

If you are bitten by a tick, your doctor may advise taking antibiotics immediately to forestall a possible infection. In many cases, however, people don't know that they've been bitten until they contract the disease. Some (but not all) Lyme-disease sufferers get a telltale bull's-eye-shaped rash, not necessarily at the site of the bite, several weeks after becoming infected. If you begin to experience joint pains and you're too young to be a likely candidate for arthritis, ask to be tested for Lyme disease.

Ask Ed Harlman, at 112 the oldest person in Iowa, why he's lived so long and he protests, "I have no advice. People keep asking me, what did I do? It gets my goat. I don't know. I can't answer that." But Ed's nurse at the Elmview Care Center in Burlington, Iowa, says *she* knows the answer: "He's just very interested in life and still keeps active. He does not sleep his life away," says Dot Smith.

Ed's zest for life makes his birthday celebration a major event at the Elmview Care Center, complete with lively music from his native Jamaica. Ed fills the role of king of the dance, loves to have plenty of people in attendance and wants everybody to have a good time. "He's just a very energetic person who loves people," says Smith.

8 | Sound Mind

Have you ever started a project at work that you were intensely interested in at 1 p.m., then—before you knew it—it was 6:30 p.m.?

Ever find yourself in such a great mood that almost no bad news could bring you down?

In a crisis, have you ever kept your wits about you when all about you were losing theirs?

If you answered yes to any one of those questions, you've experienced the incredible power of a sound mind.

No one doubts the mind's immense power to take the body for a quick spin around the block. Just sit down with a Stephen King thriller and see if your blood doesn't race or your nerves don't jangle. By "directing" your mind, Stephen King can scare the heck out of your body—whether you're reading at home alone at night or on a sunny, crowded beach.

Or listen to your favorite comic—Billy Crystal, Whoopi Goldberg, Jay Leno—and what happens? Your muscles relax, tensions drain from your body, your heart gets a workout, and the yuks cause your brain to release beneficial opiatelike substances called endorphins.

The short-term effects of the mind-body connection are obvious. It should be no surprise, then, that your everyday frame of thinking can have a profound impact on your physical life over the long haul, too. Indeed, researchers are building a mountain of evidence showing that mental well-being can improve your health and add years to your life. For example:

• People who don't reach out to others in times of stress and who withdraw into themselves suffer a greater incidence of cancer and suicide, according to a long-running Johns Hopkins University study begun in 1946.

• One in seven people who let severe depression go un-treated commits suicide. Suicide is the eighth-leading cause of death in the United States, claiming more than 30,000 lives per year.

• People with an angry and hostile personality run a higher risk of heart attack, according to research at Duke University Medical Center.

• Optimists develop fewer chronic diseases of middle age than pessimists, according to a study of graduates of the Harvard University class of '42.

• People who don't have close friends, are unmarried and who avoid community involvement are twice as likely to die than more sociable folks, according to Yale and University of California at Berkeley researchers.

This research is only the tip of the iceberg. Here's how you can tap your brain and think yourself to a long life:

85 | Recognize That Stress Is a Killer

One of the most valuable life-lengthening steps you can take is to reduce excess stress in your life; indeed, stress reduction is a common theme running throughout many of this chapter's recommendations for developing a sound mind.

Of course, you cannot eliminate all stress. Without stress, life would be dull, monotonous and, well, lifeless. The body's response to stress is as old as life on the planet itself and is intimately connected with survival. When our ancestors encountered the stressful stimulus of a saber-toothed tiger, the instantaneous rush of adrenaline and other stress-response chemicals in the bloodstream made the difference between life and death.

But while the threat from saber-toothed tigers is history, modern man's stress response remains. And our "fight or

ornelius Bode—or "Corny," as he's known around
Maple Manor in Osage, Iowa—believes his good
sense of humor over the last 102 years has been a
major contributor to his longevity. Volunteers at his
home say Corny approaches everything with a positive
attitude and is ever on the lookout for laugh lines. He
jokes about the good times and the bad. "When I sold
my farm [in the 1970s], I emptied the corn bins for
95 cents a bushel," he deadpans. "Soon as I did that,
corn went to $2.50 a bushel," he says with a laugh.
Corny also thinks having a few close friends helped
extend his life. Why, do you think? "We got together
and shared a good sense of humor," he says.

flight" biological defense mechanism is good at finding plenty
of modern threats—large and small—to detonate a reaction.
Research shows that these stressors can accumulate in the
body, lead to mental and emotional problems, and make the
victim more susceptible to illness, disease and accidents. Some
experts estimate that two-thirds of all illnesses and deaths
before age 65 are stress-related.

A stressful life and mindset can wreak havoc on your body
and manifest itself in a wide variety of ills, including heart
attack, stroke, stomach ulcers, asthma, gastritis, menstrual
disorders, ulcerative colitis, angina, irritable colon, increased
blood pressure, duodenal ulcers and headaches.

Why? Psychoneuroimmunology researchers are finding
that the brain, the immune system and the body's other biological systems continuously communicate with each other
biochemically. In response to emotions, the brain produces

substances called neuropeptides, which set off reactions in the immune system and other body systems. Those systems, in turn, can communicate back to the brain by secreting their own chemicals.

That means negative thoughts and emotions can produce clear adverse physical effects. If you can reduce the stress stimuli that produce those negative thoughts and emotions, you can reduce the damaging shocks to your body.

86 | Learn to Identify Sources Of Excess Stress in Your Life

Review a typical week to spot what things give you high anxiety. Stressors in one category—situational—are usually easily identifiable: Contact with an implacable boss, the press of rush hour, arguments with your spouse, paying the bills, opening the front door and finding your in-laws there for a surprise visit.

A second category of stressors involves self-defeating thoughts: "If I speak before a large crowd, people will laugh at me." "I'll never get the raise I want, because I don't really deserve it." "I just know I'm going to make a big mistake, because I'm a loser."

Conditional stressors make up a third category: when tight scheduling or a specific lineup of events requires you to rush out of work, run to catch your train, race home to pick up a child at school, then hightail it to a second job. Or you might have to meet a can't-miss deadline at work and make a doctor's appointment on the same day—April 15, Tax Day.

Yet a fourth category of stress is created by transitional but major life events: death of a spouse, divorce, getting fired, mortgage foreclosure. Happy major life events can also create high stress: adjusting to a new baby, moving, changing jobs, getting married and retiring. Table 8-1 lists transitional life events and rates the levels of stress they introduce into your life.

87 | Eliminate or Modify The Stressors in Your Life

Once identified, stress causers can be attacked and eliminated. For example, if you make a daily mad dash to work the way O.J. Simpson runs through an airport, you may be able to cut stress simply by leaving home half an hour earlier. A never-pleasant boss can be "eliminated"—switch jobs.

If self-defeating mental messages are the source of your tension, it would be worth your while to dig down for the hidden roots of these ill-advised beliefs to determine how you acquired them. We learn many inappropriate adult behaviors in childhood by watching and imitating the inappropriate behavior of friends, parents and other people we look up to. We also learn from sometimes hard experience. For example, a child who always gets yelled at for asking questions or who gets branded as a pest can learn not to be assertive. He may also find a rationale for the mistaken belief that "my needs are not important."

Psychotherapy or insightful self-help books and audio tapes may help you unlearn destructive beliefs and inappropriate behavior.

Some stressors, of course, won't disappear, but they can be altered. For example, reschedule commitments to uncrowd a harried schedule. Don't do the monthly bills at the end of a workday in which you've already had it up to here; plan to do them when you're more relaxed and have the energy to steel yourself for the unpleasant task.

88 | Learn to Cope with Stressors That Can't Be Changed

If you must be subjected to a stressful situation that can't be changed, you must learn to cope with it. A salesperson who can't or doesn't want to leave sales but regularly runs into difficult customers can learn techniques to defuse unpleasant situations. Putting yourself in the other person's shoes, for example, may reveal a very real customer frustration that you can easily solve. Sometimes just letting the savage beast know you're truly listening and understanding can have a calming influence.

Advance planning is another way to better cope with known stress agents. When several major life changes occur back-to-back, research shows that your chances of developing a stress-related illness can increase by 50 percent to 80 percent over the ensuing two years. Knowing this, if it's possible for you to space out major life transitions, you can have more time to adjust to one before tackling the next. For instance, if your spouse, close family member or close friend has just died, avoid making a major job change, selling the house and moving or suddenly opting for early retirement.

Table 8-1 | How Stressful Events Affect Your Life

The following social-readjustment scale has been used for 25 years to help people rate how much stress they're experiencing in their lives. Add up the numbers listed for life events you have experienced within the last year. If you score more than 200, you have a 50 percent chance of becoming seriously ill from stress; a score of 300 or more raises your chances of illness to 80 percent.

Life Event	Points
1. Death of spouse	100
2. Divorce	73
3. Marital separation	65
4. Jail term	63
5. Death of close family member	63
6. Personal injury or illness	53
7. Marriage	50
8. Being fired	47
9. Marital reconciliation	45
10. Retirement	45
11. Change in health of family member	44
12. Pregnancy	40
13. Sex difficulties	39
14. Having a baby	39
15. Business readjustment	39
16. Change in financial state	38
17. Death of close friend	37
18. Change to different line of work	36
19. Change in number of arguments with spouse	35

Life Event	Points
20. Mortgage large in relation to income	31
21. Foreclosure of mortgage or loan	30
22. Change in responsibilities at work	29
23. Son or daughter leaving home	29
24. Trouble with in-laws	29
25. Outstanding personal achievement	28
26. Spouse begins or stops work	26
27. Begin or end school	26
28. Change in living conditions	25
29. Change in personal habits	24
30. Trouble with boss	23
31. Change in work hours or conditions	20
32. Change in residence	20
33. Change in schools	20
34. Change in church activities	19
35. Change in recreation	19
36. Change in social activities	18
37. Small mortgage in relation to income	17
38. Change in sleeping habits	16
39. Change in number of family get-togethers	15
40. Change in eating habits	13
41. Vacation	13
42. Christmas	12
43. Minor violations of the law	11

Reprinted from *Journal of Psychosomatic Research*, Vol. 11, 1967, Holmes and Rahe, Social Readjustment Rating Scale, with kind permission from Pergamon Press Ltd., Headington Hill Hall, Oxford OX3 OBW, U.K.

By the same token, if you know you're headed for even one major event—divorce, marriage, new baby, new job—be prepared for the added strain and take steps to lessen the impact; for example, talk with experienced parents and spouses to learn about the trials and tribulations of parenthood and spousehood so you know what to expect.

An organized lifestyle is another great stress reducer: Establish a budget and get your household finances in order. Schedule appointments and get-togethers in a datebook. Employ lists to prioritize and accomplish daily tasks. And make sure there's a place for everything in your house and that everything is (usually) in its place.

89 | Deal With Chronic Hostility

Hostility and anger are the blood brothers of stress. Transient anger is dangerous enough, because it can lead to unexpected violence, as witness common-enough highway shootouts between drivers who have "assaulted" each other with poor traffic manners. But chronic hostility has been shown to be a killer.

No anger should be banished. Bottling up this powerful emotion is like plugging up the fumarole of a volcano; sooner or later the pent-up energy explodes forth—often with greater intensity. So anger must be dealt with by channeling it into less destructive directions.

Research by Meyer Friedman, the California cardiologist who discovered type-A behavior, shows that behavioral counseling for hostile people reduced their chances of recurrent heart problems and death by 45 percent. Professional psychotherapy can help you here, but you can also help yourself by hunting down the subconscious source of your anger and then changing your attitudes.

Chronic hostility springs from the mind – boil-overs boil down to deep-seated cynical mistrust of others. The super-market checkout boy – you automatically reason without a shred of evidence – *of course* was trying to gyp you when he rung up that carton of orange juice twice! And that darn pedestrian taking forever to cross the street in front of your car – she just wants to make you wait. And you know why a co-worker got that plum assignment instead of you; the boss is OUT TO GET YOU!

Recognize these thought processes and try to see the illogic that frequently supports them. Why, for example, would some supermarket cash-register clerk pick you out of hundreds of people to intentionally pull the old ring-up-the-orange-juice-twice trick? And that pedestrian could certainly have a lot more fun if she really wanted to make you wait for her to cross; she could stop to tie her shoe halfway across, she could place a board with nails in it on the road in front of your tires, or she could pick up a rag, wipe down your windshield and ask for a quarter. Now those kinds of shenanigans would slow you down but good!

If this strikes you as funny, you've found another tool to deal with anger: Laugh at the situation, laugh at the ridiculous illogic of your anger and laugh at yourself for concocting the heart-harming story line. If you can find the humor, angry tension can be siphoned off in the form of laughter. After all, that's the clinical definition of laughter – the sudden release of tension arising from the surprising recognition of the absurdly incongruous. Editor/author Norman Cousins helped his battle against a life-threatening form of arthritis by screening as many funny movies and laughing as often as he possibly could. In the end, he noted that laughing contributed significantly to his regaining his health.

As for your boss, well, he may indeed be out to get you. But don't get mad and don't even try to get even. Instead, try to analyze the situation from his perspective. The attempt to "get you" may be your boss' clumsy way of trying to send you a message that he's not pleased with your performance. Instead of blowing up, you may need to do better work or approach your employer to discuss potential problem areas.

Carrie Bosma is still smart as a whip at 102, and she knows exactly why she lived so long: "Because I was ornery," she says. "I always picked the berries on the other side of the bush, never wanted to do what other people were doing. I just wanted to do things differently." Carrie thinks her close friendships led to a long life too, especially the one with a childhood friend Pearl. "I've had many other close friends, but never like Pearl," who she knew until her death in her 30s. "We shared confidences good and bad, had fun together. I don't know what exactly made her special other than her way, just being Pearl," she remembers fondly.

Carrie, the Iowa individualist, devoted herself to teaching and never married. Years later, she helped run her brother's farm in Texas until he died, then she moved back to the Hawkeye State. Her advice for young folks who want to live to 100: "Live out the day you're in now; don't worry about tomorrow, and forget yesterday."

Dealing directly with the target of your hostility can help deactivate your anger, as long as you work constructively, not destructively. Ironically, your own fear of being direct may be part of the problem. Or avoiding direct discussion could be creating misunderstandings and erroneous assumptions. In approaching a source of frustration, avoid being accusatory.

Put yourself in the other person's shoes. Maybe the guy who cut in front of you on the highway is in as much of a rush as you are, maybe he didn't see you or maybe he's just a careless idiot. An offense doesn't always mean you've been specially selected for rude treatment.

Finally, don't make mountains out of molehills. Keep track of what gets your goat, then imagine the same thing happened to someone else. You may find that the same "major crime" that has befallen you would seem insignificant if it landed on the other person.

Hard as it may be for some hostile people to believe, as Friedman's research shows, you can stop assuming the worst and become more charitable in giving people the benefit of the doubt if you are committed to working at it. Try assuming the best about people and you may be surprised how many people actually live up to that standard; many even rise to the challenge just to get the approval they subconsciously suspect you'll give them.

90 | Laugh

Just as negative mental influences like anxiety and hostility can have a detrimental impact on your body, so, too, positive thoughts can produce beneficial effects on your physical being. As we've said, one of the best of these elixirs is a good sense of humor.

What's that? You say you're no Arsenio Hall? You say your jokes are about as well received as a three-days-dead monkfish in August? No sweat, because like Norman Cousins, you can buy all the laughs you need – comedy movies, TV shows, compact discs, joke books, cartoons in the newspaper, stand-up-comic videos, MAD magazine.

By continually exposing yourself to funny matter, you can develop a good sense of humor. Keeping the company of up-beat, funny people can also help you hone your comedic talents. Clipping cartoons and writing down laughable personal experiences add to your repertoire.

91 | Sing

Music is another way to restore an embattled psyche. Children's television host Fred Rogers says that as a child he banged out his anger on a piano; he now uses music on the "Mr. Rogers' Neighborhood" program to help children get in touch with and express their feelings.

Music therapists say music can alter your mood and body for the better by employing something called the *isomoodic principle*. To do this, you first listen to music that matches your mood: If you're pumped up and fed up from a long day at work, turn on the sonic opiate of angry youth – some good hard rock or heavy metal. After several songs from that genre, begin the transition to a music more appropriate for your target attitude – a soothing classical selection, perhaps, or some laid-back jazz or New Age.

92 | Be an Optimist

Humor and music help you release tension, rejuvenate your senses and put you in a more optimistic frame of mind. Studies by Martin Seligman, Ph.D., a psychotherapist with the University of Pennsylvania, suggest that an upbeat outlook on life can boost the immune system, strengthen resistance to cancer and heart disease, and promote general good health – essential ingredients, all, to a long life.

Here are our important keys to a happy, optimistic life:

• Share your life with someone you love.

• Believe in a power greater than yourself.

• Never let go of the child within you.

• Find an occupation you absolutely love.

• Stay actively involved in life and living.

• If you retire from one job or occupation, begin a new job or interest to take its place.

• Lead a balanced life, with an appropriate mix of work and play.

93 | Be a Do-Gooder

If optimism and high spirits have beneficial effects on the body, what about one natural extension of being a pleasant person – doing good deeds for others? The answer is yes, altruism is good for you, according to a study by Harvard University psychologist David McClelland. He showed subjects a film of Mother Teresa tending to the sick of Calcutta, then analyzed their saliva. He found an increased presence of immuno-globulin A, an antibody that helps fight respiratory infections.

That research, taken in conjunction with studies showing the ill effects of hostility, social isolation and stress, suggests that a giving heart can glow with health. Just reflect on your own moments of genuine generosity and recall how you felt; most people describe it as a good feeling. Imagine what it would be like to have that warm feeling all the time.

Look for opportunities to do good in the world. The trick is not to be charitable because it is a requirement. Do it because you want to. Search the catalog of life's suffering and injustices and zero in on those that you feel in your heart must be alleviated. Then find ways to make a difference.

Does a child in your area need money for a lifesaving bone-marrow transplant? Making a larger-than-expected contribution might do the job, but better yet, you might want to contact the child's family to find out how you can assist with fund-raising activities. Have you read a newspaper story about someone braving a major life crisis or do you know someone personally in such a situation? Write a note of encouragement or offer to pitch in and help.

You don't have to save the entire world from calamity to do good. Sometimes you can have a major impact by alleviating seemingly minor, everyday suffering. Take, for example, an elderly neighbor. Most of the activities and chores you engage in without a thought can be major obstacles for older people. Lend a hand! Shovel snow from your senior neighbor's sidewalk in winter; take him to the grocery store and help bring the supplies in; offer to paint her house; invite him over for a cup of coffee – or bring the coffee and some baked goods over to him one day.

You don't have to look far to find a good cause. Be creative. If you still have a tough time finding a needy cause, however, consider getting involved with more formal do-good organizations. Volunteer at the local United Way, Boy- or Girl Scouts, senior-citizens' home, area agency on aging, or hospital. Many find plenty of demand for their altruistic spirit by simply joining an organized religion or by becoming part of a good political cause.

94 | Spot and Treat Depression

An estimated 35 to 40 million Americans suffer from a major depressive illness sometime during their life, according to the National Foundation for Depressive Illness. As mentioned earlier, a depressed, pessimistic outlook on life is an assault on the immune system. Major depression can remove the very will to live.

Unfortunately, this mental disorder often goes unnoticed. Sufferers themselves may think they've just got the blues or that their depressed outlook is a sign of personal weakness, so they don't seek professional help. Those who do seek help must overcome the medical profession's seeming inability to recognize the symptoms of depression; half the time, family doctors miss the diagnosis altogether. Many depressed people see four or five physicians or psychiatrists before one diagnoses the problem correctly and begins an effective treatment.

How do you spot major depression? Don't confuse it with routine unhappiness, sadness or disappointment—"the blues" that everyone experiences from time to time and which doesn't last more than a few days, if that long. Don't confuse it with grief from the death of a loved one, either.

Rather, according to the American Psychiatric Association, major depression is characterized by the presence of at least five of the following symptoms over a two-week period:

• A depressed mood most of the day, nearly every day

• Sharply diminished interest in all or mostly all pleasurable activities most of the day, nearly every day

• Significant weight loss or gain

• Insomnia or excessive sleep nearly every day

• Agitation or sluggishness noticeable to others almost every day

• Fatigue nearly every day

• Feelings of excessive guilt or worthlessness

• Indecisiveness or inability to concentrate nearly every day

• Recurrent contemplation of death or suicide

Of course, diagnosing major depression is much more complicated than checking off symptoms on a list. For example, all of the above symptoms can show up in a person grieving the loss of a close family member or friend, and such a condition may be considered normal, uncomplicated bereavement, not major depression. Depression can be mild, moderate or severe, or it can be part of another mental or physical disorder. And major depression can take place in just one episode or be recurrent. If the above symptoms describe you, however, you should bring your suspicions to a medical professional who can apply additional diagnostic techniques.

95 | Recognize the Many Forms Depression Can Take

Depression can take on other forms, as well. Manic depression, or bipolar disorder, is characterized by large mood swings from a highly elevated mood (including such symptoms as psychomotor agitation, pressured speech, elation and flight of ideas) down to deep depression.

Cyclothymia is a chronic mood disturbance lasting at least two years, during which the person is never without depressed or hypomanic symptoms for more than two months. Dysthymia, or depressive neurosis, involves a depressed mood for most of the day on most days (rather than nearly every day) extending over a period of at least two years.

Seasonal affective disorder is a form of depression that appears only at certain times of the year, usually in the fall or winter. Situational depression is a prolonged episode in reaction to a disappointment or loss.

Research into the causes of depression has produced inconclusive results thus far, but researchers are establishing a biochemical connection involving norepinephrine and serotonin levels in the brain. Genetic links to bipolar disorder are also being established.

What can be done about depression? The most important thing you can do is recognize the symptoms when they show up—in yourself or in your loved ones. Understand that depression is not a personal failing: It is a disorder that warrants attention and that can be successfully treated. Don't be victimized twice by attaching a stigma to your depression; look at this mental anguish as though it were an unexplained physical pain and seek professional help.

The number-one reason Peter Grauer, of Marcus, Iowa, has lived so long is that he has devoted his life totally to the Lord. "You have to live every day to give God glory," the 100-year-old says. Consequently, he's always led a clean life, remained a man of strong principles, taught Sunday school and was continually involved in church work.

The Lord has taken care of Peter, too. When Peter was 86, his entire body was run over by a tractor, including his head, which was pushed face-first into the earth by the heavy wheels. The only damage Peter suffered was a small broken bone in his foot.

After that, Peter decided to expand his lifelong pursuit of music to include learning to play the piano. "Next to the word of God, music has been the most important thing in Peter's life," says his daughter-in-law. He played duets and recitals but has never failed to begin a session with the hymn "God Himself Is Present."

96 | Get Help for Depression From the Right Source

You can employ a number of self-help, mood-lifting techniques to get you out of a rut, but we recommend professional help. Some self-help remedies are likely to be part of the professional treatment of the disorder anyway, but you should nevertheless treat depression as seriously as any physical disorder and get help from a pro.

Your family doctor is probably not experienced enough to do more than refer you to a psychiatrist. Either a psychiatrist or psychologist should be capable of diagnosing your depression. Either should also be able to provide psychotherapy services to address the mental roots of the problem. But only a psychiatrist, who is a medical doctor, can prescribe antidepressants or other appropriate medications to address a biochemical source of the malaise.

97 | Heed the Warning Signs Of Suicide

No mind-based problem goes more directly to the issue of longevity, or lack thereof, than suicide. It is the emergency mental disorder—no different from a stopped heart, stopped breathing or a profusely bleeding arterial wound—and it requires immediate first aid.

Recognize the warning signs of a potential impending suicide attempt, whether in a loved one or in yourself:

• The most important signal is any communication suggesting suicide, threatening to take one's own life, or referring to how things will be different "when I'm gone." Actual attempts –"accidental" overdoses or the self-infliction of bodily harm, for example–are attempts to communicate suicidal intent. Never disregard them or assume the threats are only a joke.

• Persistent thoughts of suicide

• Withdrawal from others, a strong desire to be alone, disinterest in formerly pleasurable activities

• Symptoms of a depressive illness

• A major life crisis, trauma or loss of self-esteem that could trigger suicide

• A sudden change in personality, such as a generally reserved individual who inexplicably becomes agitated and more of a risk taker

• Bequeathal of very important possessions to friends or family members

• Sudden increase in risky activity, such as high-speed driving, carelessness, involvement in violent or aggressive behavior, or substance abuse

When these signs show up, seek professional help at once. Contact your local suicide hotline or consult your family physician or a psychologist or psychiatrist.

Know who is at greater risk of taking her own life. Suicide is the second leading cause of death among people ages 15 to 24. Too, for people age 75+, the death rate from suicide is about twice the average for all ages.

98 | Jettison 'Old Baggage'

"Old baggage" is a popular psychology phrase that refers to all the unresolved conflicts and burdensome beliefs that everyone has banging around in their heads. Have you never been able to openly disagree with your mother? Are you absolutely terrified of taking a chance and falling flat on your face? Do you get hooked into ridiculous arguments with your spouse because you need to prove you're head of the household?

It's all Old Baggage that should have been repaired or discarded long ago. Worse, unless you perform a mental housecleaning to get rid of this stuff, you end up carrying every piece of this baggage wherever you go. That can weigh down anyone. And like excess physical weight, excess psychological pounds can shorten your years.

One of the most obvious ways in which unresolved issues reveal themselves is substance abuse. Experts know that people who abuse alcohol, drugs, food or any substance are trying to medicate and protect themselves from the pain of this excess baggage. The drug-induced stupor or the folds of fat become a wall behind which the abuser can safely hide from his mental anguish.

Likewise, compulsive behavior can protect its victim from powerful fears: The compulsive saver may be building a wall of money against deprivation; the workaholic may find safe refuge in being the master of her work because she fears the risk of intimate human relationships; the obsessive gambler may be trying to prove – to himself and everyone else – that he really is a winner, not the loser that his mind keeps accusing him of being.

To keep these mental handicaps from cutting years off your
life, you need to recognize and resolve your feelings of guilt, low
self-esteem, jealousy, suspicion, hang-ups, shyness and fears.

Any number of books dedicated to each specific problem
can help you understand and get over these stumbling blocks.
Psychotherapy can also help you learn more about your
thought processes and correct troublesome misperceptions,
erroneous beliefs and self-defeating attitudes.

Research at the University of Pittsburgh's Cancer Institute
suggests that flushing out destructive thoughts can be a real
life preserver. Two sets of patients whose cancer was in remis-
sion received different treatments – either standard medical
care or psychological training to develop coping techniques,
learn relaxation and nurture optimism. The patients with the
psychological training developed more active natural killer
cells which guard against new tumors.

99 | Get Married, Get Friends

For years now, more and more studies have shown that
married men and sociable women live longer than single men
and keep-to-themselves women.

For more than 30 years, the Duke Longitudinal Studies
have observed three groups of people: men who connected
with more friends, women who attended meetings of various
kinds, and men and women who withdrew from social
activities. People in the first two categories were happier and
healthier than those in the last category.

The world was not a very warm and caring place when Gertrude Clay, of Selma, Alabama, came into it on January 6, 1892. Born on a Southern plantation, she's endured more than her share of hardship and injustice. But her mother and her grandmother, who was blind and had worked in slavery, taught her to live life according to the Bible. Gertrude has followed that guidance her entire life and still quotes the scripture at 100. And she says *that* is the secret to long life. "The Lord gave me the privilege to live so that I could serve Him," she says.

Doctors might conclude Gertrude's ways have reduced stress and prevented anger from poisoning her; philosophers would surely say she has found inner peace by becoming one with the world. But Gertrude offers a more down-to-earth homily: "Live a good life, be kind to people, be faithful, trustful and honest. For all the good you do, God blesses you."

Other studies have found that friendship brings more than just well-being; they show that the risk of death is lower for people with friends and spouses. For example, research done by the Survey Research Center of the University of Michigan showed that the death rate for more reclusive women was 1½ to 2 times greater than for more social women. Men in the same study who were involved with few friends and activities had a 2 to 3 times greater chance of dying.

And researchers at the University of California at San Francisco have shown that unmarried men and women between the ages of 45 and 64 were twice as likely to die within a 10-year period as their married counterparts.

Does this mean a confirmed bachelor or bachelorette should run out and get married? Not necessarily. The life-stretching benefits of marriage and friendship are related to marital status but seem not absolutely dependent on it.

Married men fare well, the experts say, because of the nurturing they get from one of the wife's traditional roles as caregiver. Wives also tend to be a positive force pushing husbands toward healthier habits and nutrition.

But by far the most important element marriage and friendship provides is interconnectedness with another human being. After his wife dies, a widower tends to grow depressed, gets sick more easily and his overall health can rapidly deteriorate. Consequently, in the first several months of widowerhood, men have a greater propensity for following the wife into the grave than widows have for following their husbands. Researchers say the culprit seems to be the man's grief over the loss of his only soulmate.

Widows and widowers behave differently. The men, for whom the wife tends to have been their only confidante, retreat into loneliness and suffering in solitary confinement. Widows, on the other hand, who often have a circle of close friends beyond the husband, turn to them for comfort and consolation, and to share their problems and fears.

Too, according to the UCSF study, a person who simply lives with another gains nothing in longevity over the married person; she runs the same morbidity risk as an unmarried person—probably because the commitment between roommates is decidedly different from that between two people who have decided to journey through life together "until death do us part."

Bottom line: Marriage definitely provides life-extending benefits worth seeking, but that relationship should be buttressed with a number of additional close friendships.

Rush Limbaugh Sr. is needlessly apologetic about the fact that he's missed work recently because of bouts with pneumonia. But that solid work ethic may have been this 100-year-old Cape Giradeau, Missouri, lawyer's fountain of youth. "By all means," he says without question, "keep working. Stay busy. People with the health, will and desire should work."

Rush long ago overruled any motions to retire. "I never wanted to retire, because if I did I would've disappointed a lot of clients," he says. The selflessness of that remark—the idea of working for the benefit of others, not solely himself—indicates another possible secret to Limbaugh's longevity: giving, loving, family-oriented values.

Rush, grandfather of national talk-radio personality Rush Limbaugh, became a member of the bar in 1916 "because lawyers help keep order in society. I enjoy court work and the excitement of taking a case through to see if I can get the right thing done." He married his childhood sweetheart, Bee—"The best thing I ever did; she was a great companion and helpmate"—and remained close to the home and family he and Bee established. He also found time to pitch in at local hospitals, his church, and the Boy Scouts.

Rush also has advice on what not to do: "One of the most damaging things in the world is to get angry and work with that anger inside you. I've always tried to be friendly, keep my cool and work that anger out of my system."

100 | For Men Only: Think Like a Woman

Professor Henry Higgins – the ever-perturbed *My Fair Lady* character who asked, "Why can't a woman be more like a man?" – would die to hear it, but maybe he had it backward: Men should be more like women. If living to 100 is the game, women know something men don't. On average for all races in the United States, women live about seven years longer than men. That numerical edge is roughly the same throughout the industrialized world. The hormonal advantages of estrogen in women and the disadvantages of testosterone in men may explain some of the disparity, but not all of it.

Men, however, start out with a statistical biological advantage: At conception, male fetuses outnumber females by about 115 to 100. By birth, the ratio is 105 male, 100 female. At age 30 the numbers are even at 100. From there, females build an impressive lead that, by age 80, gives them a late-game ratio of 50 males to every 100 females.

The last thing we want to do is step into the crossfire of the war between the sexes. So, herewith, we present – without further blasphemous comment – a brief compendium of statistics that might offer some worthwhile insight:

• The top-10 leading causes of death – heart disease, cancer, cerebrovascular disease, accidents, pulmonary disease, pneumonia, diabetes mellitus, suicide, liver disease and atherosclerosis – all kill men at roughly twice the rate they kill women.

• A study of bomb-ravaged London in World War II found that 70 percent more men than women became psychiatric casualties.

• Men are murdered three times as often as women.

• Men smoke, drink and engage in risky practices at a greater rate than women.

• Men are more likely to drive after drinking and have twice as many fatal car accidents per mile driven as women.

• Women suffer depression at about twice the rate of men, but male schizophrenics outnumber the female kind two to one.

About the Authors

Charles B. Inlander is president of the People's Medical Society and has been its executive officer since its founding in early 1983. He is co-author of more than a dozen books on health care. Mr. Inlander is a faculty lecturer at the Yale University School of Medicine, and his articles have appeared in scores of publications. Prior to joining the People's Medical Society, he was an advocate for the rights of handicapped citizens and the mentally retarded. A native of Chicago, he is a graduate of American University in Washington, D.C.

Marie Hodge is a senior editor with *Longevity* magazine. A longtime health and consumer reporter, she has written for *American Health, The New York Times, New Choices for the Best Years* and *New York* magazine. One of her cover stories for *New York* won the National Magazine Award, the most coveted award in magazine journalism.